Chubby Gal Fitness

Weekend Exercise Getaway

July 2012

Hi Grandma,
I hope you enjoy the book I wrote.

I love you!
Wendy

Wendy Strack

outskirtspress

DENVER, COLORADO

Chubby Gal Fitness
Weekend Exercise Getaway

Cover Photo © 2012 JupiterImages Corporation. All rights reserved - used with permission.
Author photo credit to Ford T. Pearson, www.ArtofFord.com

Outskirts Press, Inc.
http://www.outskirtspress.com

ISBN: 978-1-4327-8792-9

Outskirts Press and the "OP" logo are trademarks belonging to Outskirts Press, Inc.

PRINTED IN THE UNITED STATES OF AMERICA

Dedicated to my husband, Clayton, and my family.

Table of Contents

Introduction

I decided to write Chubby Gal Fitness because it seemed like a fun thing to do for a gal who's about twenty pounds overweight. Keeping a healthy weight has never been a problem until marriage, a comfortable life, and a desk job caught up to me. I knew it was coming but I can't say I resisted too much while it was happening.

I am a chubby gal who lives in a rural area on the outskirts of Hells Canyon. During the week, I drive over an hour one way to my job, put in eight and a half hours, come home and take care of chores on sixteen acres. My husband, Clayton, helps tremendously when he's not out of town working for months on commercial vessels or research boats as an engineer. On a typical work night, I unwind from my long drive by cooking dinner. When Clayton is home, we use this time to chat about our day and then eat around 9:00 p.m. before turning in. I know, this is so bad! But we enjoy it. Out here when it's time to work, it is *time to work!* So, on the weekends we dine out, watch TV, and do absolutely nothing if the opportunity presents itself. The extra weight I put on was caused by me and I did it to myself fair and square.

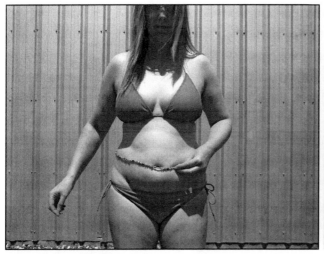 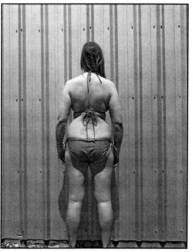

Mind you, I am not interested in losing weight on purpose at this moment. If it happens it happens, but it won't be a result of careful planning. I have planned so many times that I'm not into it anymore. Life happens and life couldn't care less how much I invest in meal planning and exercise programming. The last weight reduction program I started ended after a brush with poison sumac. My arm was dripping with blisters for a month and planned exercise, even modified, was not an option. Another failed attempt at weight loss was during the summer, when friends invite friends to impromptu gatherings where food and drinks take center stage. I could only say no to the neighbor's invitations so many times before I began to act like a skinny bitch. No one wants to keep inviting a skinny bitch to their party. People gather and eat and that's not going to change. People are getting bigger and we are reminded of this every day.

I did not write Chubby Gal Fitness to lecture and tell you you're going to die if you don't get the fat off. I'm not trying to change the world and I am not out to help you lose weight to save your life. There's no tough love here. If you're healthy and moderately active but only have time say, on the weekend, to squeeze a little exercise in then you are going to love this book!

It's Not About Losing Weight

If Chubby Gal Fitness isn't about losing weight then what's the point? Why write a fitness book for chubby gals and not promote weight loss? That's weird.

I'm glad you wondered. Read on.

I believe words such as 'long term goal', 'measurement', 'outcome', 'protocol', 'program', and 'competition' are relics from textbooks written by and for a long lineage of Club Jock members. Those of us who are not athletes tend to associate exercise with working out and chubby people work out to lose weight. Working out is synonymous with discipline, (something athletes have but apparently not people trying to lose weight), and discipline is required if you are desperately trying to stay afloat on a long term program. Workout, discipline, and program make a chubby gal like me want to go hide in a closet. I don't know about you but the terms relating to exercise sound so severe they don't inspire me to even want to move. This is a problem. Compounding the problem is the vicious cycle of counting calories, falling off the wagon, getting back on the wagon and falling off again. And again. How can anybody feel good doing that? It's no wonder bingeing has evolved into a favorite pastime since the activity truly imparts a warm and fuzzy feeling.

If you are bent on losing weight and think you need a barking personal trainer kicking dirt at your heels, then I say settle down and hang out with me for a weekend instead. You will get a wonderful variety of "workouts" and you might even like the idea of exercising when it's all said and done. What I am bringing to the table is a whimsical package full of warm fuzzies rather than relics. There will be a constant change of scenery from a variety of venues, there's cheap entertainment, interesting trivia, good grub, and oh yeah - exercise! Not boring exercise-by-rote but themed exercise to keep you interested.

As a potential bonus, exercise can lead to better fitness. And that will come in time as you exercise more frequently particularly on weekends. After all, fitness is the ticket to enjoying a vast and rugged playground like Hells Canyon. It is through this book that I invite you to my home and 'hood where your weekend exercise getaway can be vicariously fulfilled. Which brings me back to my point. Becoming an active player in a world spilling over with recreational opportunities is more important than beating yourself up in the name of losing weight. Chubby Gal Fitness weekend exercise getaway is where it's at and you are so there!

Start Where You Are With What You Have

I realize most people reading this book do not have access to a designated national recreation area with wild and scenic rivers and wide open spaces and you might not even own dumbbells or a jump rope. Don't let this stop you from moving that body of yours. As you will soon find out there are plenty of good quality exercises within these pages that you can do with limited space and equipment. In addition, I offer different activities that may be suitable to how you're feeling toward exercise at certain times. For example, if you just want to hang out and aren't really interested in doing a shuttle run or bike ride then do mat exercises. If you're feeling hyper and don't have the patience to focus on proper form or technique, let go and dance. There is nothing written in stone with any of the exercise sessions because this is not a book about programming. It is a book about ideas you can play with according to what you have, where you are fitness-wise, and how you feel at the moment.

Now, oddly enough, there are some chubby gals who might think they can't start exercising until everything in their world is perfect, including their bodies. It's kind of like tidying your house before the cleaning lady comes to *clean it*! Sounds crazy but you just gotta start on the fly and leave everything as it is. Kind of like going away for the weekend. In the end, everything will be fine. Exercise, even for a little bit, lets your body experience the deliciousness of being in its natural state. Your mind, with all its overanalyzing and thoughts of perceived barriers, will pick up on the positive energy resonating from an active body. Next thing you know, your mind will be more willing and less resistant to physical activity.

But you have to start! It's that being in the moment thing. Doing something now with what you have *now*.

The Way I Roll

Exercise is not something that should be forced. Like me, some people may not have grown up in an athletic environment. I enjoy exercising on my own terms but I ebb and flow with regard to consistency. If I go for a jog it's because I want to. When I pick up a dumbbell it's because I want to. Many times I don't count reps and sets because, well, I don't want to. When I get off the couch or out of the kitchen it's when I want to. Not when I'm supposed to simply because a schedule is staring at me from the refrigerator door. The schedule usually gets ignored anyway. If nothing else, exercising needs to done as an act of pleasure. This is easy to achieve when you adopt the mindset of a hedonist by going to an exotic location, whether for real or in the imagination, and picking whatever pleasurable physical activity appeals to you.

There may be some types of exercises demonstrated in this book that you find attractive and others not so much. You know what? That's ok! I don't like activities where balls fly at my face. Volleyball, softball, and baseball turn me off in a hurry. I still have nightmares about playing for a grade in college when I really, *really* did not want to. You see, when I was a kid I was walking down my street and didn't know a mischievous neighbor boy had hidden behind a wood fence. He flung a rock at me for fun and nailed my head with it. I never even saw it coming. When I got to my house I was a dazed, bloody mess which freaked my mom out. If that wasn't bad enough, I had to get stitches for the first time ever. Many years later, when I was albacore fishing commercially, the taut line I was pulling in lost a fish. As a result, the jig flew out of the water, hurling itself at mach speed, coming to an abrupt stop only after ricocheting off my face. I have never experienced such stinging throbbing pain in my life! Long story short, I understand if there is a physical activity you would rather avoid than participate in. So I made it a point to present you with options to explore without too many iron-fisted rules. 'Cuz that's the way I roll.

I Ain't Your Momma!

I am childfree by choice which means I'm not a mom. Call me a fitness enthusiast, tour guide, hostess, cook, entertainer, (well I try!), and writer but don't call me mom or late for supper. Since I ain't your momma, don't do anything you do not feel safe doing. Let common sense prevail and nobody gets hurt. After all, we aren't in it to win it. We are on a weekend getaway that just happens to involve exercise. Bring a sense of humor and some curiosity but most importantly, relax and have fun with this stuff. With that said, there is a safety meeting overview in the upcoming paragraphs. Hells Canyon isn't called Hells Canyon for nothing, you know.

Safety Meeting Overview

Among one of the many hats I wear is safety coordinator. Here's a little somethin' somethin' to make sure your active stay, (remember, you're living vicariously!), is a happy one:

1.   REGARDING HELLS CANYON

Hells Canyon is big! Big heat, big rivers, big waves, big wildlife, mammoth cliffs, and isolation in grand proportions. Rugged wilderness for the adventure-minded woman can be dangerous but it can also be big fun. Preparedness and a healthy awareness of your surroundings in my backyard will help you enjoy and not regret your visit. Enjoying the surroundings is super fun and super safe with a buddy. Know where you're going and let others know when to expect you back. Pack minimal gear for comfort and safety including a hat, sunglasses, hairclip or band, tissue in Ziplock bag, sunscreen, lip balm, water, snack, foghorn or whistle, and snake bite kit. It's not a bad idea to add flashlight with fresh batteries, forceps, knife, 1st aid kit, meds, and a two-way radio if you plan on getting lost for a while. (That's a joke). Seriously though, if you think you're going to be gone for more than a few hours take the extra gear just in case. Safety, comfort, and good times with friends are priceless.

2.   REGARDING EXERCISE

The exercises in this book are not tricky. Some are quite common. Challenging? Sure. Tricky? No. You won't find me nagging constantly about perfect form. In fact, you can't even see your form half the time anyway, like in a T-push up. I am not making it my job to nitpick you to death. Your body with all its wisdom will guide you away from harm but you have to listen to it. No one knows your body the way you do so listen to and respect what it's signaling. Nevertheless, whenever you begin an exercise session it doesn't hurt to start with simple calisthenics like jumping jacks, marching in place, rebounding, or jump roping for a few minutes. This will cue the body in on what it will soon be doing and give you an opportunity to avoid potential injury.

It is a safe bet to assume that whatever position I show you, you would mirror. I throw this out there because I don't guarantee all of the instructions start with something proper like, "stand with your feet shoulder-width apart, knees bent at 90-degrees." If you see me standing, sitting, laying on my back or belly, then my position speaks for itself. If you see I'm standing then I will (sometimes) save you the burden of having to read it. Suppose I am standing but also bent forward from the hips. Does this mean you squat? No! You bend at the hips also. Chubby gals are smart and they get it. Yes, I do offer coherent instructions but it's not always textbook.

There are many ways for a chubby gal to modify physical activities to match her current fitness level. No matter what a gal does she needs to make sure any health issues are under control. If you are dealing with an acute condition just enjoy the scenery, cheap entertainment, trivia, and recipes for now and save exercise for another day. Let the scenic photos within this book inspire you until you are able to exercise safely. If you have uncontrolled chronic health issues, ditto. If you plan on jumping in with both feet then great! I've got your back with exercises that can help improve overall conditioning. Because I am somewhat of a rebel, I left out numbers of reps and sets since those will be determined by your personal fitness and strength levels. How much you do is up to you.

3. REGARDING EXERCISING IN HELLS CANYON

The main thing is to get all hot and sweaty without killing yourself. Don't get so dehydrated that you end up delirious and forget where you're at. Remember, this is Hells Canyon baby! Prevent sunburn, avoid heat stroke, don't put a bunch of beef jerky in your pockets and decide to follow a trail to a cave full of carnivores looking for shade. That would be bad for both of us! Check out Appendix B: Some Safety Stuff for more information regarding your safety in my backyard. It's pretty interesting and it might even save your life.

Chubby Gal Weekend Getaway Itinerary

Friday, AM for most of the day:
- ✓ Scenic jet boat tour into Hells Canyon National Recreation Area to Hells Canyon Dam, returning to Heller Bar. Box lunch provided.

Friday, PM:
- ✓ Arrival to Tiki Hut Lounge. Dinner and cocktails.

Saturday, AM:
- ✓ Outdoor Adventure in Chief Joseph Wildlife Area. Breakfast and lunch provided in the field.

Saturday, late afternoon-early evening:
- ✓ Midday R & R to include foot soak, dog care, crafting, target practice, baking and canning, among other things.

Saturday, PM:
- ✓ Recovery Rave with snacks and beverages.

Sunday, AM:
- ✓ Working Homestead with breakfast.

Sunday afternoon:
- ✓ Final Departure.

CHAPTER 1
Getting Here is Half the Fun

Friday, AM for most of the day:

Whether you drove a little or a lot or flew in on Alaskan, Horizon, or Delta to my friendly hometown airport, your weekend getaway starts with a scenic jet boat tour from the Hells Canyon Marina in Clarkston, Washington. You will be greeted dockside by your personal captain, Tom, who happens to be my neighbor. His girlfriend, Laurie, will be your hostess. The *TNT* was built in neighboring Lewiston, Idaho, the jet boat manufacturing capital of the world. Not only is Lewiston the only commercial port in the entire state of Idaho but nearly all the great rivers in the Northwest come to, through, or near Lewiston. The twin cities Lewiston-Clarkston, also known as the LC Valley, sit at the mouth of Hells Canyon, which is the deepest gorge in North America. And you are going there!

Once Captain Tom checks that everyone has arrived and is on the boat he will start the powerful dual Corvette engines, cut loose from the dock and navigate through the Snake River Reservoir. Laurie will provide whatever music you want to listen to on the premium sound system. If the late morning air seems chilly, don't worry one bit. In a matter of time you will experience pockets of heat. The deeper you travel, the more frequent the pockets, until it pretty much feels like the inside of a convection oven turned up high.

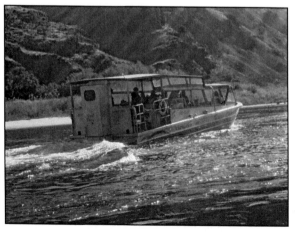

The reservoir offers a festive atmosphere with jet boats, jet skiers, water skiers, pontoon, and sailboats buzzing all around. As you head out of town on the *TNT* you might also notice the locals walking, jogging, and riding bikes on miles of paved levee pathways. You may even be neck to neck with commercial jet boats or even a working U.S. mail boat full of tourists. The mail boat follows an historical route on the river to deliver news and parcels from civilization to remote ranches.

In the 1880s, there was a short-lived homesteading boom. Settlers threw in the towel after they realized how much they had to battle the weather to farm and ranch. However, some ranchers still operate today. Thus, the need for a working mail boat.

Guess what? You're going there but you won't have to deliver any mail! Meanwhile, I will be floating downriver on a raft or racing on a jet ski with Clayton and our friends until rendezvousing with the *TNT*.

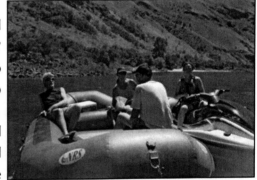

Hey, I see the *TNT* coming now and there you all are! Do you see me waving? Tom does so he slows down, allows me to board then keeps cruising at a steady clip because we have a lot of ground to cover.

"Hello, hello!" I greet my weekend guests. After introducing ourselves and drying myself off, I take a seat on the cushion bench inside the cabin. The landscape begins to take on a more remote tone although the river continues to parallel a well-used road. Basalt layered hillsides carpeted with brown grass flow down to the riverbanks where scruffy trees, beaches, and green grass decorate the river's edge. Although there are many people recreating on the water and beaches, there is a ton of space and room for everyone. The *TNT* travels at a leisurely pace for a few good miles then slows down. I get my guests' attention as we pull up to an historical site.

"The first part of our sightseeing tour begins at Buffalo Eddy," I say. I point to the right where a large white beach is dotted with tents, campers, and dogs frolicking about.

"There's a short paved trail from the road that leads you to rust-colored petroglyphs. Pre-Nez Perce tribes drew them over 4,500-years ago," I say. "We aren't going to stop today but you will have a chance to come back tomorrow during the outdoor adventure segment. Right now we have a lot more to see upriver!"

Tom keeps moving for a long stretch before slowing with caution. He steers clear of approaching six foot standing waves in the middle of the river known as Captain

Lewis Rapids. Talk about a wild water tantrum!

"Ladies, about the time you think civilization has turned into complete remoteness is the time you come to Heller Bar," I inform them. Once again, I point to the right.

"As you can see, this public access lot fills up with trucks, boat trailers, rafting camps, and motor homes. This is *the* hot spot on the Snake River for bank anglers who travel from all over to fish right smack here!"

Trucks with boats on trailers are lined up at the ramp to get their boats in the water. The parking from Heller Bar overflows on to the road above it. Immediately beyond the craziness of Heller Bar is the mouth of the Grande Ronde River.

The Snake River got its name in an amusing way. There was a miscommunication between the first white explorers and natives from the Shoshone tribe. The explorers watched the natives make an S-shaped movement with their hands to represent swimming salmon. The explorers probably did not know what a salmon was and mistook the gesture for a snake. The name Snake stuck instead of Salmon. Nevertheless, one of the three largest tributaries flowing into the Snake does happen to be the Salmon River.

"The Grande Ronde means large valley," I say. "The river originates in Oregon and terminates here at the Snake."

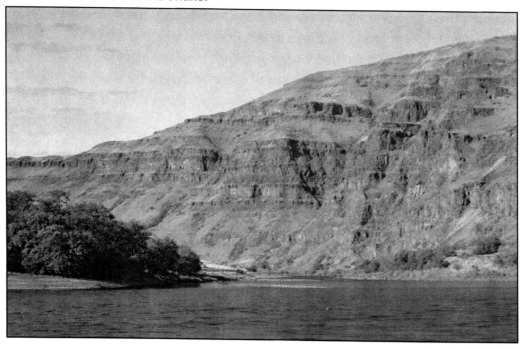

"Off of the tributary and on the Snake River bank is the town of Rogersburg," I add. "Rogersburg is small. There are probably fewer residents living there than there are kids in a third grade classroom, it's that small. Rogersburg remains the farthest upriver access point by vehicle and is the only place north of Hells Canyon dam where you can drive along the river in Oregon, Idaho, and Washington. Another interesting fact is that Rogersburg is sitting on a couple buried caches. Maybe you'll be the ones who find them?" I tease.

The ladies smile. I continue.

"This area which includes Heller Bar, the Grande Ronde River, and Rogersburg, is where we'll be returning after the Hells Canyon tour. Your weekend will mostly take place on the Grande Ronde and Snake Rivers. You will also be in the Chief Joseph Wildlife Area which is part of the Grande Ronde River," I explain. "Now, I'll be quiet and let you enjoy the boat ride into Hells Canyon! Oh, just so you know, there is no cell phone service out here."

The *TNT's* loud, powerful engines rev up enough to put the kabash on talking anyway. Meanwhile, Tom gets us out of civilization where there are no more roads along the water. Even so, there is an amazing amount of river activity with jet boats and rafters, white sand beaches with campers and volleyball nets set up, as well as quaint weekend cabins built on rockier beaches. The cabins are well cared for and modern with the exception of outhouses and generators. The beaches where the cabins reside look like jet boat central. Rows of colorful boats rest with their bows on the sand, tied off while people party on them, in the water, on the sand, in the cabins. The people wave, we wave back. Tom keeps going and we soon find ourselves coming into a more solitary and pristine environment. To the river's right appears an oasis in the middle of arid, hilly landscape. The *TNT* slides next to the dock, gets tied off and off we go. As we walk on the trail I inform the gals where they are.

"Ladies, you have left the state of Washington and are now in Oregon and Idaho territory where you will remain all the way to the dam. This here is Cache Creek Ranch. You have officially entered into Hells Canyon!"

Amongst the oohs and aahs are raves about the sheer beauty. The gals follow a path to lawns and an abundant fruit orchard. Because of the shade, birds are plentiful and deer are present. Tourists always love snapping a few shots of the wildlife. My gals have a chance to learn a bit about the canyon's natural and cultural history which is explained on exhibits inside the house. The canyon was originally called home to the Nez Perce people, who wintered here due to the mild temperatures. White people changed all that in the late 1800s and early 1900s. Homesteaders and businessmen stepped in. Try as they might, sheep and cattle ranchers, and prospectors barely scraped by. Most flat out went bust. On the other hand, Cache Creek Ranch thrived as a sheep ranch in the 1930s. Now it is an administrative site staffed by a facility host.

"Pendleton wool came from this area," I say. Then ask, "who's ready for lunch?"

We gather at a picnic table with individual boxed lunches placed on it. Herbal iced tea in mason jars are set next to the boxes. Lunch consists of vegetarian falafel pita sandwiches, sides of chilled cucumber-mint raita, lentil salad, and a lemon bar. Perfect fare for a hot summer day in Hells Canyon.

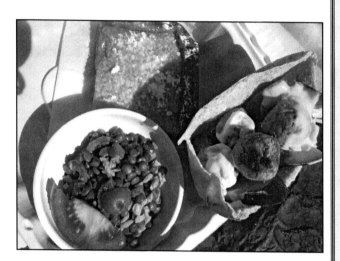

About caches. It was common practice for natives to store food such as dried salmon at river crossings. A pit was dug by the women where they placed extra food in baskets or handcrafted hide bags. They then covered the cache with earth and marked it with rocks to come back to at a later time.

After lunch, we collect our items and make sure to take one last pit stop before loading onto the *TNT* where the voyage continues.

"Keep your eyes open for mule deer, bear, bighorn sheep, elk herds, river otters, mink, golden and bald eagles, blue heron, and water fowl," I say. "At night, hawks, owls, bats, skunks, raccoons, porcupines, coyote, and fox come out of the woodwork. If you're lucky, you might get the chance to glimpse a bobcat or cougar during the twilight hours. That's always exciting!"

One of the ladies fans herself with a magazine.

"It's getting hot," she says.

"I know. And it's only going to get hotter. You'll have a chance to swim, I promise!"

Twenty miles from Heller Bar and coming at us from river left is the mouth of the Salmon River. Owning the nickname, The River of No Return, the message is clear.

Only skilled and experienced operators should navigate it. Because of its free-flowing nature and constant current, the Salmon has been a popular floating destination with rafting companies.

"The Salmon River flows freely for over four hundred miles," I inform the ladies. "For as long as it is, it remains in only one state. Idaho. There aren't any other rivers in the lower forty-eight that can make a claim like this."

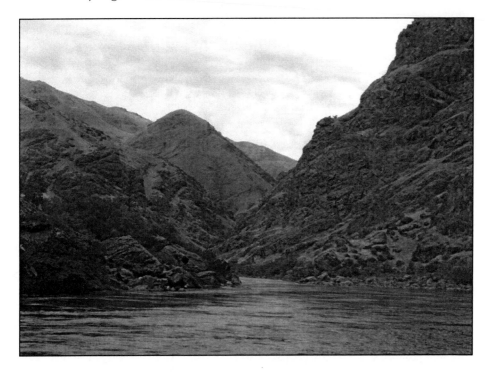

There is a four mile distance between the Salmon tributary upriver to the rockier Imnaha tributary. Tom makes a pass through Imnaha rapids near the mouth of the Imnaha River on our right. The composition of the cliffs takes on a more jagged texture which imparts a sense of going deeper into wilderness territory. Remnants of old foundations, tiered rock walls, a railbed, and tunnels unfold within this short stretch where the mill town called Eureka used to be.

"Just above the confluence, a mine tunnel over 700-feet was cut across the ridge," I say. "Entry into the tunnel is gated off to protect people and the endangered big-eared bats who call the tunnel home."

Tom locates a beach and carefully runs the bow of the *TNT* into the sand.

"You may go swimming now," I suggest. "The water temperature is probably seventy degrees. Enjoy!"

And we do. While in the water, I point low on the mountain wall.

"Do you see the iron rings there?" I ask. "Paddlewheel ships of the 1900s needed to use cable lines to help pull through the rapids. They didn't have enough power on their own. One sternwheeler, the *Imnaha,* sunk after a line got caught in the wheel. It turned sideways in

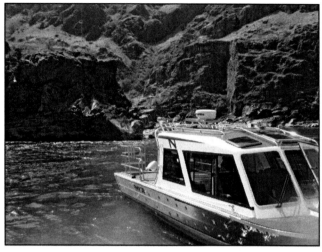

the rapids and died here," I say. "All the passengers were saved. Unfortunately, a prize white stallion drowned."

After a delicious excursion in the cool grotto, we board the *TNT* for more adventure. Dug Bar is the next destination where Tom brings the *TNT* to the beach. Here, in the middle of nowhere, is a small concrete boat ramp and an airstrip. Nearby, an interpretive site sadly tells of Chief Joseph's Wallawa band of Nez Perce Indians making their forced river crossing to the Lapwai Reservation in 1877. Two thousand U.S. Cavalry was no match for the natives so elders, children, horses, and cattle traversed the high and fast water flooding with spring runoff. Chief Joseph would never return to his land.

In a moment of silent reflection our party continues to pass through one of the deepest parts of the river at Deep Creek. The Snake River depths can be as low as two to three feet to over one hundred. Cache Creek and Deep Creek are about one hundred five feet to river's bottom.

> **Long before white man came** to homestead and seek out their fortunes, the Nez Perce (Ni Mi'i Puu) were the authentic stewards of this region, home to wild and free flowing waters.

"In 1887, a band of outlaws tortured over thirty Chinese miners for their gold in this part of the canyon," I state. "Bodies tossed in the river floated to Lewiston which is how anyone knew anything even happened. Although there were men who got caught, no one was ever punished for the massacre."

A change in scenery comes in the form of distinctive columnar basalt at the river level. It looks like someone carved tall vertical steeples into the rock wall. In contrast, the geological tapestry also includes pillow basalt that could pass for elephants on the beaches and hippos in the river. Throw in some craggy breccias and all you can do is shake your head in awe.

Pittsburg Landing is next on the Idaho, or left side, of the river. This is one of the rare road accesses where vehicles can drive down to the river within the gorge. Located on a bluff above the river with high peaks rising on all sides was once an expansive Native American village site. Today, it is a campground where remains of ancient civilization past still exist on rocks marked with pictographs and petroglyphs.

"As we continue our journey, we will be passing through the oldest rocks in Hells Canyon," I inform the gals. "The vertical jagged walls you're looking at are over 300 *million* years old! This is probably the most dramatic border in the country, with the mighty Snake River drawing a deep, serrated line between Oregon and Idaho."

> **At lower elevations along the** streams are abundant deciduous bushes and trees. Sagebrush, bunchgrass, prickly pear cactus, and poison ivy are prolific, as well. Western larch, Douglas fir, and ponderosa pine inhabit midway, while spruce and sub-alpine fir top off the highest elevations.

"This isn't the place to explore with a motor home, that's for sure," one of the gals remarks.

She is right. Hells Canyon offers an intensity and rugged severity matched by few places in the United States. Sheer cliffs reach for hundreds of feet to the heavens, dwarfing everything in its devilish shadows. In fact, Nez Perce Indians named the gorge, the Place of Shadows. Hidden within this place of shadows, on a narrow, flat bank is Kirkwood Ranch. The *TNT* cuts through large roller coaster waves at Middle Kirby Rapids approaching the historic ranch. Once again, Tom brings the boat to the bar of land that had been farmed and ranched from the mid-1800s until 1974. That's when the government turned this site into the recreation area it is today. Full time hosts working two month shifts live here.

Everyone in our party wanders the green lawn, with some of us sticking our feet into the cool, swift creek that has a churning waterwheel. In the museum and interpretive sites, we read about the family who lived here, in the deepest part of Hells Canyon during the 1930s. Kirkwood Ranch was the first house in the canyon to have a bathtub. That was living the high life! Less than a mile up from the ranch was another cabin called the Carson Mansion. The high life was being lived here also.

"The Carson Mansion is known as the Moonshine Mansion," I say. A few gals hike with me to check it out. The simple structure isn't near what one might consider a mansion by today's standards.

"It's so small," a gal observes.

After we reload on the *TNT*, I lead the ladies to the stern and point at a hazy cliff side under a bright blue sky. There is an obvious horizontal scar.

"That is Suicide Point, a trail carved in the cliff 400-feet above the river," I say. "The trail is single file and, believe it or not, sheep herders moved their flock along that trail to follow the sunflowers each spring. Pack animals and horses went too. A native named Half Moon and his horse fell to their deaths. That's not the way any of us would want to go, I'm sure!"

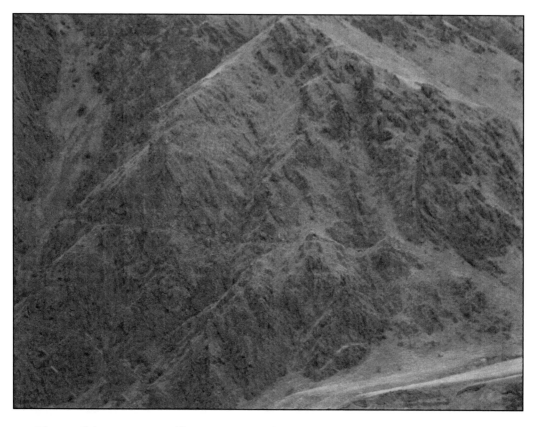

The trail becomes smaller as we travel upriver until it simply disappears from sight. A few miles ahead brings us to a river turning wild with louder and more turbulent water. Life vests are put on and not one person hesitates. The *TNT* throttles through big volume rapids that smack against the hull. Avoiding large boulders and big holes is one challenge for the captain while large roller coaster waves present another. Depending on water flows, a rock in the water at Waterspout Rapids can make a hole big

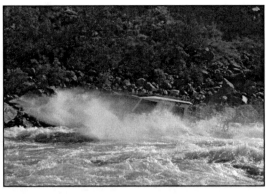

enough to eat a boat for breakfast. Today, the water is high from the dam flows, so the class 4 rapids have washed out.

The heat is heavy and overbearing. If a person were to press her hand against a rock long enough she would certainly burn it. As difficult a landscape as Hells Canyon is, there are always unexpected sights to soak in. If it isn't glazed, black river-polished boulders along the banks, or steeply dipping and folding layers of light gray limestone formations, then it is fields of gravel pits scattered about the hills as testimony to catastrophic landslides.

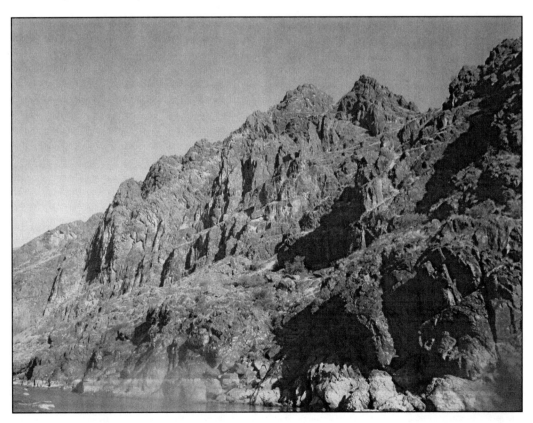

We pass gravel beaches and numerous boulders on the river right and more roller coaster rapids with even deeper troughs. Yet, that isn't enough action dished out in this neck of the woods. We have come to the most dangerous stretch of the mighty Snake and now we are committed. Turbulent, explosive, pounding, pushing, and aggressive waters are in our face, in the boat, on us. All we can do is enjoy the ride while washing machine waves full of chaos, confusion, and power try tearing us up. An enormous green wave with a deep trough breaks over the bow, creating quite a reaction. Waves continue to tangle around boulders strewn like pebbles in our path. Six miles to the left in Idaho and one-and-a-half miles vertical, is the home of He Devil Mountain, peaking at 9,300-feet above sea level. We are not quite to 1,500-feet elevation but are holding on for dear life! And then, to our right up ahead we see refuge. The Hells Canyon Recreational Visitor Center.

"We have finally hit the wall," I tell my guests. "As you can see for yourselves, we are at the Hells Canyon Dam and can't go any further. Most jet boats never make it up this far. They turn around and for good reason."

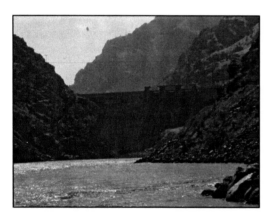 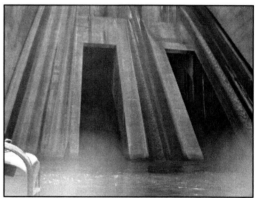

The departure off the *TNT* is made in record time with the gals scrambling to get to the visitor center. Inside, a theater, exhibits, air conditioning, and a bonus in amenities - modern toilets, are available to the exhausted travelers. One particular historic site in the neighborhood is Hibbs Ranch, known for ambush and murder that had taken place many moons ago. It is still unsolved today.

"If there are any amateur sleuths, this might be a cold case for you to investigate," I say.

Back in the day, a pioneering dad equipped his children with pistols and advised them to shoot to kill because they might not get a second chance.

After a short respite from the river, the ladies and I step onto the *TNT* one last time for the trip back to Heller Bar.

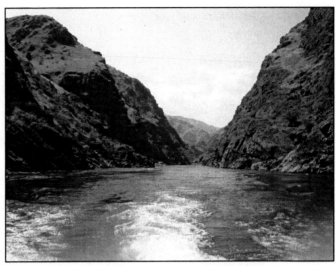

The *TNT* makes an about-face and charges through the exciting, wild river, allowing the surge to help us along. We pass a party of rafters that had put in at the visitor center launch point. They appear to be enjoying the barren landscape while drifting in a calm pool after surviving two of the fiercest rapids, also called drops, on the river.

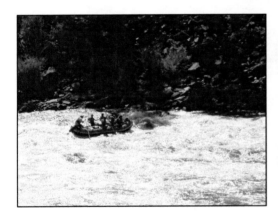
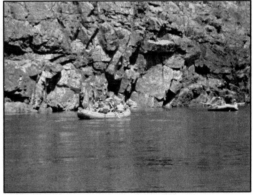

As we retrace our footsteps downriver, I fill my guests' imaginations with stories about the canyon's geology, Nez Perce tribal legends, and disappearing wooden boats. I tell tales of world-class fishing and explain where the boundaries are that make up the scenic and wild portions of the Snake River. Just about the time the chubby gals' heads are spinning, I see an opportunity for some cheap entertainment.

Cheap Entertainment: Where's the Ram?

Where is the wild ram?

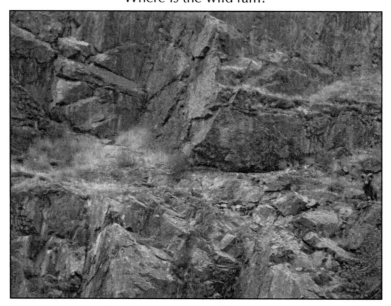

There he is!

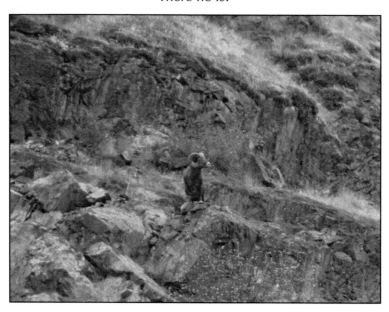

CHAPTER 2
Tiki Hut Lounge

Friday, PM:

After a long day of jet boating and sightseeing, dusk is fast upon us. Tom offloads our party at Heller Bar. Clayton and his friends are in the busy lot waiting with our transportation to the house. Grizzly ATVs and a Polaris RZR, (a utility vehicle with side by side seats), are going to take us there.

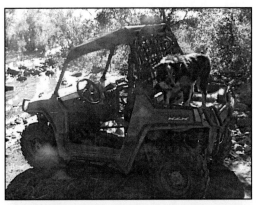

I lead the group on one of the rigs a few miles along the Grande Ronde River. We get dusted out a time or two when vehicles come from the opposite direction but the warm breeze feels good. Chukars and partridges scatter about when they see us coming. We slow down where wild sheep and rams stand in the road. Some aren't in any hurry to move and the gals love it. A few moments later we arrive at my *hacienda* on the hill.

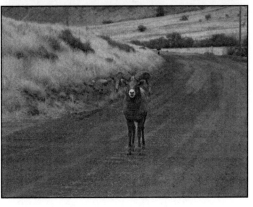

My weekend guests settle into their rooms for a chance to freshen up before coming out to the patio to mingle at my private oasis called Tiki Hut Lounge. Tiki Hut Lounge is both a covered patio lounge and my exercise studio, which is enclosed but can open up to let the outside in.

Tiki symbolizes a primitive way of life where it's okay to sip coladas in a jungle hut wearing a mumu. All right, maybe that's a stretch but it does conjure up images of sunning, hunting for seashells, and gathering baby hermit crabs. In the land of Tiki, this truly is a productively active day. And without a doubt, it is how I like to be productive with simple leisure exercise in a simple tropical setting. But since I live in Hells Canyon and not on an island, my Tiki Hut Lounge is the next best thing.

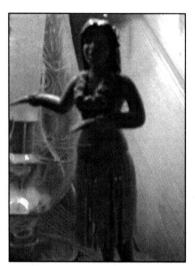 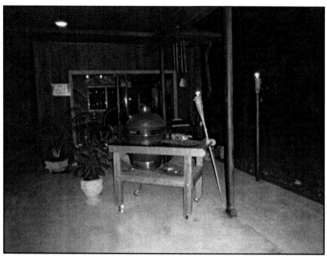

Way back in the day, I was a deckhand on a commercial albacore tuna fishing vessel. I can still recall entering through the Passe Tiputa in the French Polynesian region of the South Pacific Sea. The bow of our seafaring vessel was greeted and led by bottlenose dolphins to the inside of Rangirora atoll. There was no end in sight to the calm turquoise water. In fact, the lagoon was so large it had its own horizon. The skipper never discouraged his crew from jumping over the heavy metal rail into 85-degree highly saline seawater. Because of the saline, we were able to float and not sink while swimming around the 95-foot steel hull, frolicking in waters of paradise. That evening, the crew from our sister vessel met a soap opera star and her manager husband and invited them aboard their vessel. While everybody sat around the galley table sharing tales of adventure, the earlier day's swim came up. The soap star's eyes got huge.

"I would never swim out there!" She gasped. "My husband and I feed the sharks from our bungalow and there are a ton of them! They're all over!"

With that said, we all loaded into dinghies and went to a thatched roof lounge for drinks to contemplate what might have happened but did not. Then we moseyed to an open-air restaurant where barefoot servers brought us dinner.

The first mai tai I ever tried was on Rangirora. Ice was not a common commodity and drinks were served room temperature – warm. Apres dinner and mai tais, a Polynesian dance show capped off the evening. After all these years, there's still a little Tiki in me and I'd like to believe there's a little in all of us.

"Welcome to Tiki Hut Lounge!" I say. "No shoes? No problem! Bikini attire is the dress code so come on over!"

There are plenty of warm and chilled pu pus piled on hardwood platters.

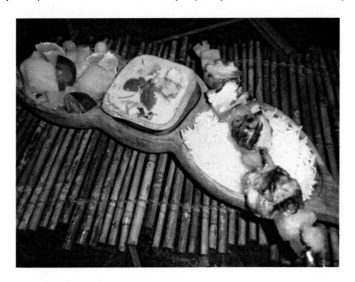

"Don't let the word pu pu ruin your appetite," I insist. "What it means is bite-size appetizers with a Polynesian, Hawaiian, or Asian flavor. In other words, exotic. Typical pu pus include spareribs, eggrolls, and fried shrimp. None of which we're having tonight."

"Oh bummer!" One of the gals replies.

"Instead, Tiki Hut Lounge is serving up organic mango with key lime halves, cod chowder with an Asian twist, and teriyaki marinated filet of albacore and pineapple kabobs on steamed basmati rice. How's that sound?"

"Awesome!" Another guest answers.

Everyone smiles in anticipation. The smoke-filled air smells breathtakingly delicious. Clayton helps me bring the shish-kabobs to gustofactory perfection on a domed-lid ceramic griller and smoker known as a kamado, also dubbed the Big Green Egg. The uber-moist tuna and pineapple bites have a hint of smokey undertone to them.

"Pu pus are for whetting the appetite before an entree, if in fact you still want a meal after nibbling on such succulent appetizers. They're supposed to be simple and light," I explain. "On the same note, it's not a bad idea to ease into exercise, especially if you've been out of the groove for a while." The ladies nod in agreement and nibble. I continue.

"Tonight's exercises are designed to get your body primed for the duration of the weekend. I planned this little sampler to be simple and light. Of course, everyone is unique and might have a different opinion of what I consider to be simple and light once the session gets under way. That's ok! What's important is to get your feet wet, so to speak. The exercises might be familiar to some yet exotic to others. Nonetheless, I think once you try a couple you'll agree this is a *swank* good time!"

We stand around chatting, nibbling, and laughing.

"It's never too late to exercise at Tiki Hut Lounge," I say. "Follow me!"

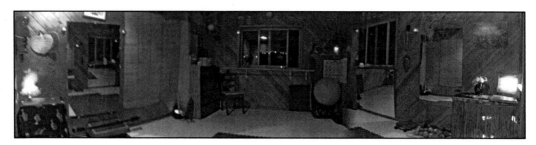

"The focus is on leisure overall toning with an emphasis on the backside of the body," I point out. "A fun and carefree warm up using a scooter leads the progression. A mat, a pair of small, light-weight squishy balls, as well as a large stability ball, and a toning bar are used in this short session. The theme appropriately relates to the seashore. Snorkeling or swimming anyone? There aren't any sharks here!"

Warm Up with Scooter

You might have a 4-wheeled scooter if you've got house plants. If you don't have plants or a scooter, or if you have issues with balance and coordination, you can improvise. To improvise, mimic the action on your hands and toes. It's not as exciting as having wheels though. More importantly, you will look fabulously silly messing around with such a thing, if you are indeed using a scooter. If scooting or improvising isn't your thing then march in place while swinging your arms. Nevertheless, you can still reap the benefits of good quality low impact movement the whole body can appreciate.

For starters, get your bearings. You can do this by shifting your lower body from the hips back and forth like a pendulum or tip-toeing as a modification. I'm not gonna lie when I say it requires effort to coordinate upper body stability, core strength, and lower body movement. That's because this isn't a move we typically do on a daily basis. It is fun and will make you laugh. Of course, you can switch it up by placing your hands on the scooter instead, with your feet, (and/or knees), on the mat to stabilize you. Or, simply sit and scoot. Whatever position you try, it's all good!

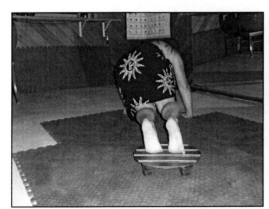 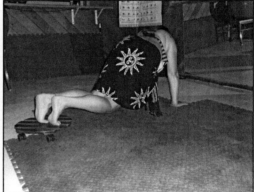

The Orca

A majestic creature with grace and strength not unlike yourself. The orca starts you off easy using only a mat. Your lower back, butt, and hamstrings will feel the work. Lay belly down on a mat with arms stretched out to the sides. Palms up or down, it doesn't matter. As you can see mine happen to be up. Your face is off the mat and so are your shoulders. Belly, hips, and thighs are in contact with the mat. Your legs are bent, knees about hip-width apart and toes touching each other. Tighten your abs and slowly raise your knees followed by the lower thighs up off the mat about an inch or so. Hold, hold, hold and release. Then do it again. And again.

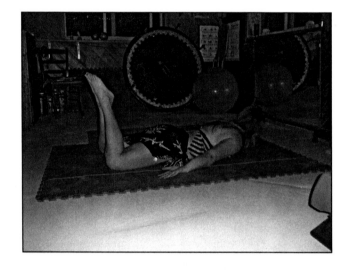

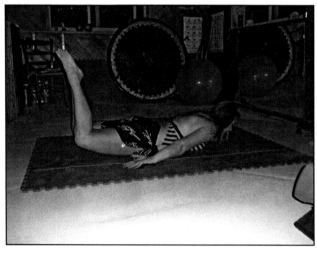

Synchronized Swimmer

Me, a synchronized swimmer? Huh! At least I can pretend with this slick move. Feel free to amp things up by adding a stability ball. I kid you not though, things get tricky when an exercise ball is resting between your feet. Your whole body goes into action to stabilize the sideways position. In addition, both the legs and core will certainly feel the squeeze. In a good way, of course! Try this without the stability ball, if you prefer.

Lie on one side placing the ball between your feet, (optional), and push up to balance on your hand. Hold as still as you can by activating your core. At the same time, you will raise your opposite arm to the ceiling as I do in the picture. Twist your upper body toward the mat and attempt to reach underneath your torso. When you've done that, return to start and repeat. Switch sides when you're ready.

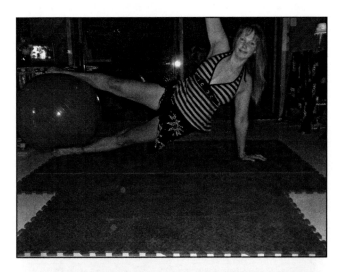

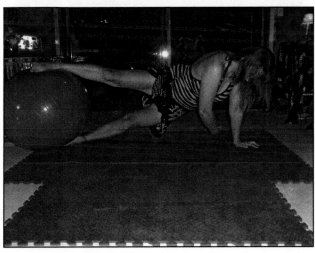

The Stroke

Continue using a stability ball for this exercise, commonly known as a sidestroke or front crawl. In addition, grasp a squishy ball in each hand. This movement uses both a pull-through and recovery phase at the same time. This is great for strengthening and loosening tight muscles in the shoulders, back, and chest. Stabilizer muscles fire up as you rest on the stability ball. You can try this without any weight at first, especially if you have shoulder issues.

Lay on the big ball, either on your torso or belly region, whichever is most comfortable. Find balance with your foot positioning while keeping your legs straight for stability. Notice my left arm extends all the way out front and my right arm is all the way back, almost against my side. Think of your arms as a windmill moving opposite each other. Pull the left arm through and below your torso while bending at the elbow. At the same time, move the right arm forward as the left arm is pulling beneath you. Continue this fluid movement. In other words, swim!

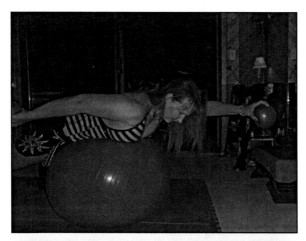

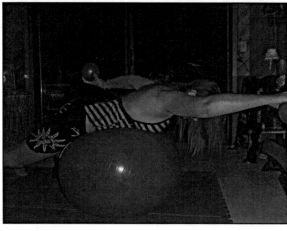

Butterfly - Dolphin

Yes, this is the butterfly but I'm also calling it the dolphin. Why not? I know you want to dive and glide like a dolphin. Who doesn't? If you were to swim the butterfly-dolphin in the water you would notice that it's a bit more challenging than the previous stroke. Since you are not in the water, the dolphin kick part of this exercise won't be executed. However, you will get the chance to kick very soon. You will be activating your upper body, both front and back muscles, by using those squishy toning balls.

What you want to do is lay belly down on an exercise ball, feet wide enough to allow you to balance on your toes. Hold your arms above your head to make a "Y". Push the arms straight back beneath your body. Arms rotate so your palms face up, at which point your arms lengthen all the way out along your sides. Keep your head up to maintain alignment. Bend your elbows slightly then rotate both arms back to the start position. Repeat.

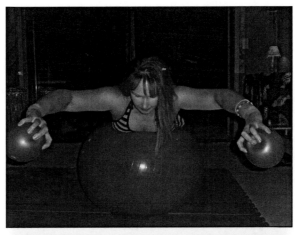

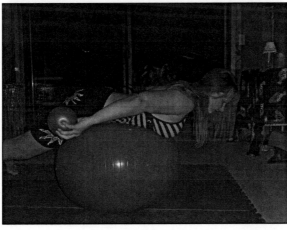

Glute Kickback

Now you can take a break from the stability ball since all you will need is the mat and one squishy ball. Since the dolphin kick was left out of the previous exercise, here's your chance to do some kicking. Well, ok, it's not really kicking but close. This glute kickback will work that bottom of yours and maybe even hamstring if you tweak it just right. If you don't want anything behind your knee, that's fine. You'll still be doing good.

Get on all fours, making sure a small ball is within arm's reach. If you use the ball, pick it up and place it behind the bend of your knee so it fits snug. Carefully extend at the hip by drawing the leg back. A contraction will, (or should), be felt in the butt cheek. Lower your leg without dropping the ball and do it again on the same side. When you've had enough with the one leg switch to the opposite leg and repeat.

Strong glutes will benefit you when snorkeling in that bikini! When you have completed this exercise, go ahead and set the squishy ball out of the way, get up and sit on the stability ball. You will also need a toning bar.

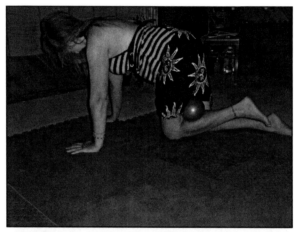

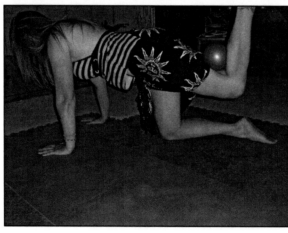

Seated Chest Press on Stability Ball with Toning Bar

Don't let the long name put you to sleep. This is a simple chest press done while seated on a stability ball. I thought it would be fun to dig out my toning bar and demonstrate something with it. That something is a front upper body move which is the perfect counterbalance to all the back work you pulled off. You will also be recruiting stabilizer muscles. If you don't have a toning bar then use the squishy balls or dumbbells instead.

Sit on a stability ball with the weighted bar in both hands. With feet on the mat and back aligned, hold the bar close to your upper chest. Tighten your girdle and press away from your chest. Slowly bring the bar back. That's it! Continue doing this until you get your fill.

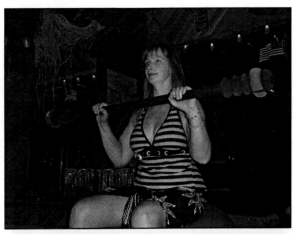

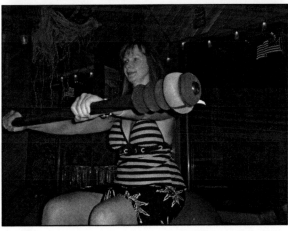

"Super job!" I praise my enthusiastic guests. "Wouldn't you agree that was just the right amount of exercise? Now, you should still have plenty of energy to enjoy what's in store for the rest of the evening. There are plenty of pu pus, Trader Vic's libations, with no shortage of ice by the way, cheap entertainment, and hot tubbing. Who doesn't love a great party?"

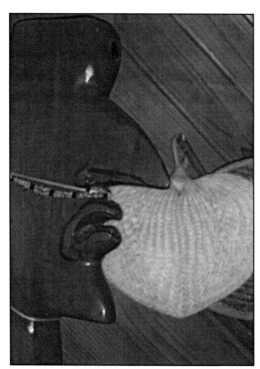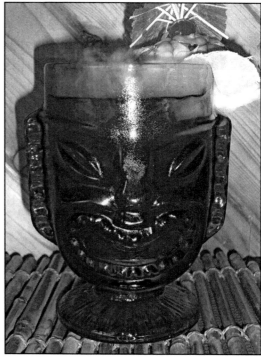

Cheap Entertainment: Coconut Bowling!

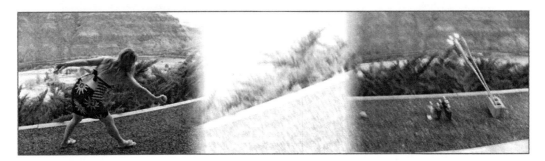

A great game to play when everybody's taking it easy. Here's how we do it at the Lounge:

The set up - Collect empty bottles and set them up like bowling pins. Grab a coconut or two and stand back at a reasonable distance establishing a foul line.

The action - Stand with your back straight, shoulders square facing the pins and knees slightly bent with both feet together. Adjust your *slide foot* slightly in front of the other one. If you're a right handed bowler you will slide with your left foot. In other words, your slide foot will be the opposite of the hand you use to bowl with. So, go ahead and place that slide foot in front just a hair.

Here are some tips you can use to refine your technique. Prior to making the first step, (by stepping out with the back foot on the coconut side), try pushing the coconut straight out until your arms are fully extended while at the same time placing your empty hand across to the coconut to support it from underneath.

As you begin your second step, let the coconut swing straight back smoothly without using too much force. Over swinging may cause your shoulders to twist toward your coconut hand and throw your aim off.

During the third step, the coconut should be on its way back forward. Remember not to apply force.

Your fourth and final step should coincide with the release of the coconut, sliding your feet forward if possible.

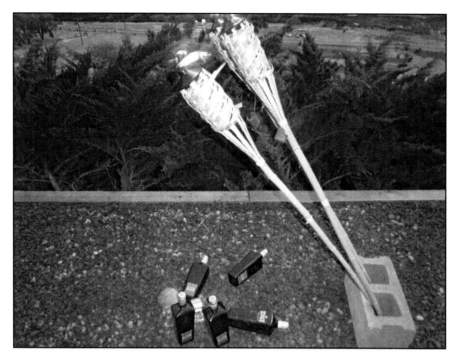

Caution! Never run to the foul line when making your approach toward the empty collection of glass rum bottles. Especially if you've been drinking rum.

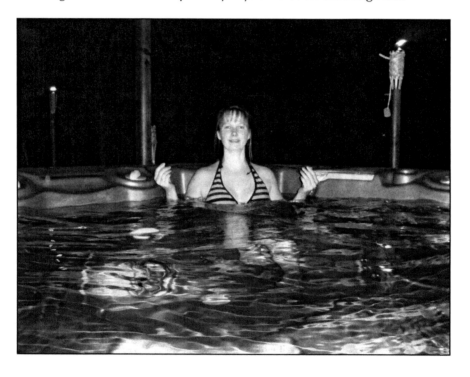

CHAPTER 3
Outdoor Adventure

Saturday, AM:

"Good morning!" I greet the gals. We gather at the top of my steep driveway. "I hope last night wasn't too hard on any of you."

"Had a great time!" One of the guests claims.

"I love hearing that!" I respond. "Today is an activity packed day. It starts with a walk to my neighbor Pollock's house. That's where we will have breakfast."

There's a look of curiosity from a couple of ladies. I smile.

"Follow me."

As we walk the unpaved road along the Grande Ronde River, rugged layered cliffs contrast with gentle beaches where a tent or two has been pitched. The sun rises above the water, creating a spectacular view.

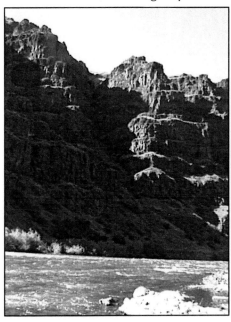 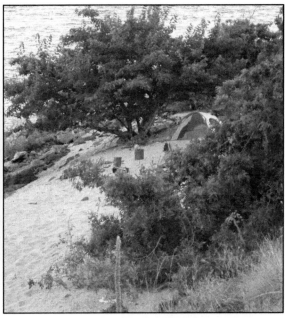

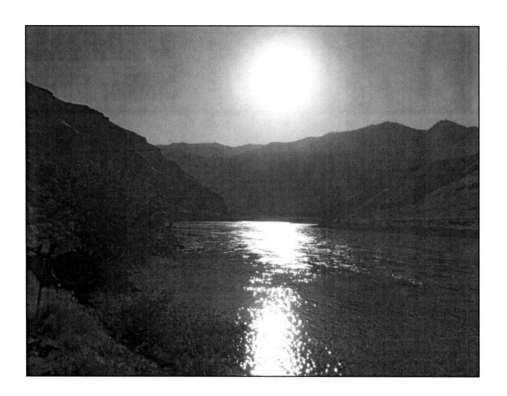

"Good, old-fashioned outdoor exercise rocks my world," I reveal. "Noncompetitive and solitary or small group activities make me a happy girl. Give me a lot of space, a bike, kayak, or a hill, and I am in my element. Sagittarius is my sign and don't fence me in is my motto.

"No matter how fancy a fitness club is, it's still not the same as being in nature," I continue. "I compare it to biting into a peach the second it comes off my tree. Sweet nectar drips all over my hand and forearm. Exercising indoors all the time is like canned peaches. They're dull and need to be artificially sweetened to make up for the fact that they are dead. This example may be dramatic but my point is clear. Outdoors is better than indoors."

The closer we get to my neighbor's beachfront yard, the more a wafting scent of meat over a campfire beckons. We follow the smoke and finally arrive at the source. As breakfast is being tended to, I offer ginger capsules, sugar-coated ginger candy chews, and coconut water to anyone who might be feeling the effects of last night's overindulgence. No one wants to admit they are hung over but I can tell. Snooki and the Situation aren't the only ones who party. People on the river know how to have a good time too!

"Ginger helps soothe an upset stomach," I say. "I'll even pack it with me if I know

I'm going on a high intensity bike ride because of all the sludge I move through my system. That makes me nauseous every time." I wander closer to the beach, where kettlebells and hula hoops are laid out.

"Who's ready for some cheap entertainment?" I ask.

Cheap Entertainment: Kettlebell Toss into Target!

If you want to feel your nervous system in action, put your hands on a kettlebell or two. Because of the off-centered weight distribution, you become aware of an automatic function hardly noticed but critical to orientating yourself in space. It is called proprioception. Proprioception is a primitive sense even more so than smell. Moving your arms or legs in a particular way without looking at them is an example of proprioception. Learning a new motor skill using kettlebells taps into this mysterious sense.

How to Play:

1. Set up an outdoor target, in this case a hula hoop and not the dog.
2. Give yourself enough distance from the hula hoop, then position kettlebells on the ground where you can reach them.
3. Squat to pick one up by the handle with one or both hands.
4. Straighten the legs and come to a standing position but keep knees slightly bent. At the same time thrust your hips upward and swing the bell to shoulder height. Allow shoulders and arms to rise and fall with the momentum.
5. When the bell swings back between your legs give one more thrust and release the bell toward the target area.
6. If you missed you don't earn any points. If you made it you get a point.
7. Run to retrieve your bell and bring it back to starting. If you scored then step farther away and toss.

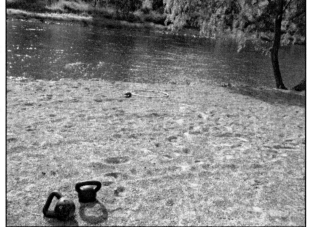

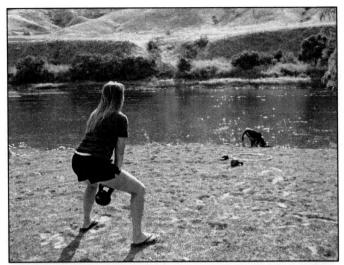

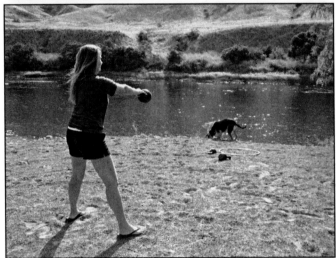

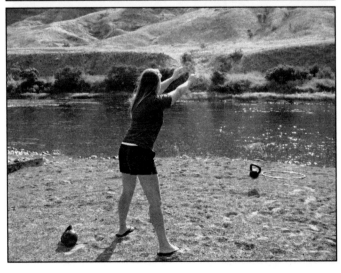

"Chow is ready so come an' git it!" The cook hollers. Three cast-iron pans go from the open flame to the picnic table. Fried sweet potato chips, eggs, and gorgeous hunks of pan-seared salmon are smoking hot. So are our appetites.

"When you're done with that, grab a big slice of granny smith apple strudel and some OJ to wash it down with," I say. "You want the energy because it's going to be a busy day!"

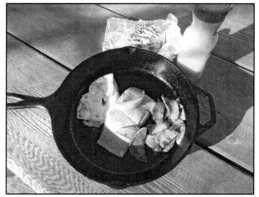

As we eat, I present the various types of activities that are to take place in the Chief Joseph Wildlife Area.

"Today you will be on, or in, two rivers and three states, depending on what you decide to do," I begin. "Here are the choices." I pull a set of notecards from my backpack and pass them around. The information highlights adventure options available to my guests.

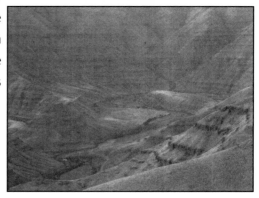

River activities: Kayaking and River Running

Kayaking, paddling, or touring is super for an upper body workout and for building core strength. That's because there is a lot of rotation from the torso when you negotiate through the water. For those with arthritis or bad knees this activity is low impact.

River running, walking, or jogging is a refreshing way to develop balance while toning the entire body. The aerobic system is used as well. By pumping the arms, keeping the core engaged, and pushing the legs against the water, you have an awesome fitness option here.

"I personally like keeping my float under control while touring for wildlife instead of white-knuckling it in class D-I-E rapids," I admit. "And for river running, I ask got river? Got dog? Got running shoes?"

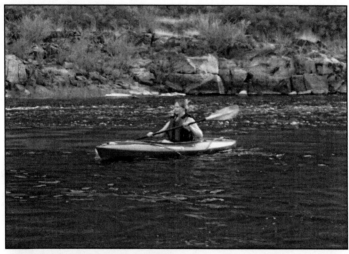

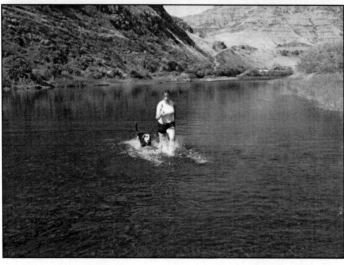

On wheels: Biking and Rollerblading

Biking requires coordination and endurance, it strengthens the lower body and tones the upper body. It even strengthens the wrists but does not stress bones or joints. The scenery changes dramatically on a bike, which makes riding that much more enjoyable.

Rollerblading uses muscles you forgot you had, like internal hip rotators. Balance, agility, speed, endurance, coordination, low body strengthening, and flexibility are reasons to get your wheels on. By swinging your arms, lower body propulsion becomes activated. Sounds kind of dangerous! If you take your time and refine your skills, this can be very exciting! Balance challenged? You might not want to try these activities until your status improves.

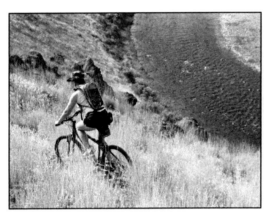 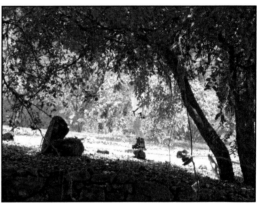

"Steep hills are a fun way to push yourself when bike riding," I comment. "Sometimes you have to get off the bike and actually push it. I do this often. When it's hot outside and my heart rate maxes out I'll end up lying on the ground to bring it back down. Otherwise, I ain't going nowhere!"

When I was a kid I loved exploring on my bike and would do it for hours. To this day, nothing feels as good as being part of the rain, sun, and warm summer breeze. As an adult, I have found there is nothing better for a sore back than a bike ride.

When Clayton and I moved to Hells Canyon many years ago, I biked alone. Not too smart since there are predators out here. Naiveté vanished after I had a chance to witness, from the safety of being inside my house, a very big cougar creeping out of my pole barn at sunrise one morning.

If the weather is mild I will take one of the dogs. Dog or no dog, I pack a loaded pistol or a mini foghorn to let whatever's hiding know I'm coming. My rides typically last an hour before I decide to return or keep going. It's hard to stop when there are homesteads to look at with acres of beautiful gardens and flashy peacocks milling about. Wild turkeys might be roosting in oddly large nests in scrappy little scrub trees or flying through a golden field. Cooler temperatures along creeks and rivers are always a welcome relief and so are the plump, tart blackberries.

When I feel rested and ready to get going again, I enjoy cruising by impressive herds of elk. They watch me watch them. This is wilderness territory and getting around out here is worth every minute of exercise. This is what being fit is all about.

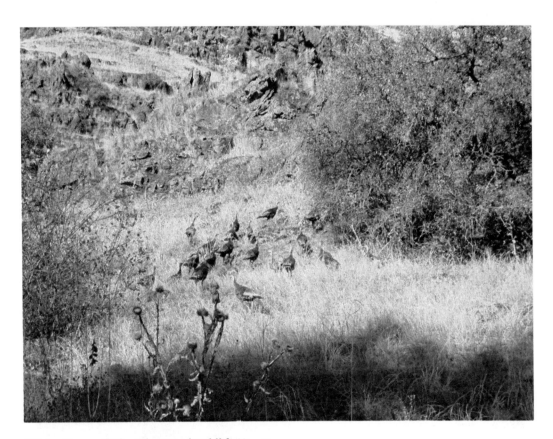

Off the Beaten Path: Hiking and Wildlife Viewing

Hiking is an activity that invites you to open your senses, take a look at scenery from other perspectives, and locate treasures that you would never know about if you hadn't hiked there. The joy comes from taking your time and not rushing past everything. You can actually be mellow and tinker around in nature's living room.

This activity hones your balance, is ideal for low impact endurance, and tones your legs and butt. Hiking is bonding time with your dog. What's not to love?

Wildlife viewing is for anyone who is both curious and patient. The payoff happens when you see deer playing tag, when you witness a baby wild sheep who mistakenly thinks she's a deer, and when watching a cougar stalk deer from a mere six feet away without ever ambushing them. Don't forget to bring binoculars and a field guide. Hiking and wildlife viewing is something anyone can do.

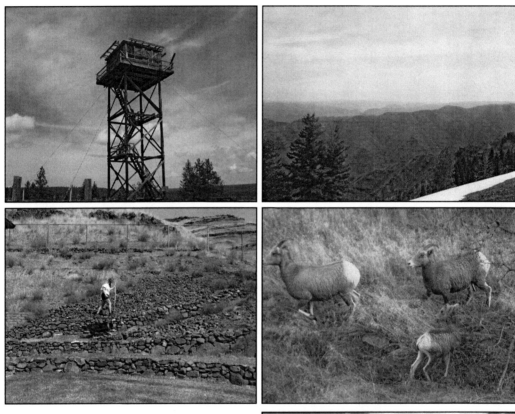

"It is hard not to get your feet wet when you're standing at the river's edge," I say. "But beware of poison sumac! This innocent looking foliage is something I would pick for a flower arrangement if one of those Martha Stewart moments came over me. Unfortunately, I didn't have to pick it because it got me anyway." I pull a few pictures from my field bag and pass it around.

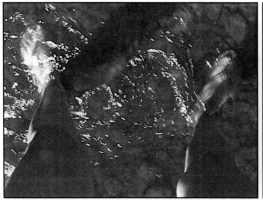
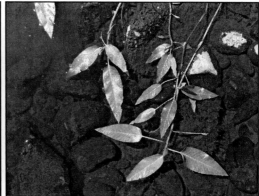

"This is my forearm dripping with blisters. I put baking soda on it to help dry up some of the moisture but there really wasn't much I could do except wait it out for a month. Let me tell you, that was not fun!"

I walk to a pile of gear on the lawn.

"Lunches are supplied in your packs," I inform the gals. "You get to eat like a twelve-year-old today with peanut butter and jelly sandwiches, energy bars, mini candies, cheese and crackers, and even some freshly plucked lemon cucumbers. Stay hydrated and keep your electrolytes up with coconut water.

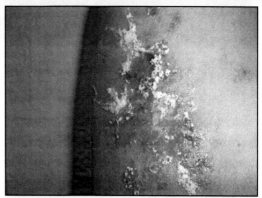

"Also provided in your packs are a set of maps for the receational activities you will be doing around here. If you need anything, just radio me or Clayton

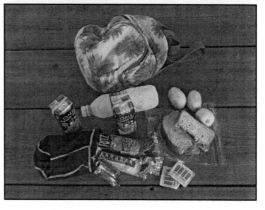

because a radio is in the pack also. An ice pack, soothing gel, and warming cream are for you to put on any sore muscles while out in the field."

Recreational outdoor activities require finesse, balance, coordination, power, endurance, and multi-directional movement. The upcoming exercises should help refine performance skills and can be accomplished with minimal equipment.

Simple stretches are always good to do before, during, and after physical activities of any type.

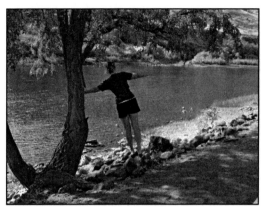 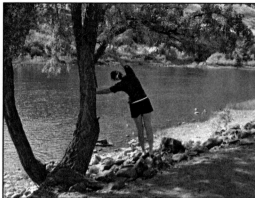

Warm Up Skipping Rope

I love skipping rope! There is nothing more rewarding than maintaining a consistent cadence without tripping over the rope and smacking yourself. It truly can be bliss. Not only is this a simple warm up but it is wonderful for circuit training and cardio. You can travel with a rope and it's real easy to skip during commercial breaks when you're watching TV. Skills of balance, coordination, rhythm, timing, agility, and reflex come as a result of skipping rope.

The instructions are simple for a basic jump. With the rope behind you, stand with your feet together and a slight bend in the knees. At the same time you turn the rope, push off from the balls of your feet. Don't jump too high, just enough to clear the rope. Land lightly with soft knees. Continue rotating your wrists while jumping *lightly*. With practice, you will be able to skip non-stop for five minutes with ease. I can go ten minutes no problem. An hour, no problem! It's like learning to ride a bike. Once your body remembers how to do it, skipping rope becomes second nature.

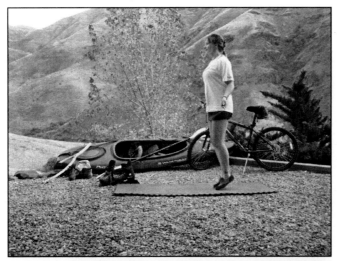

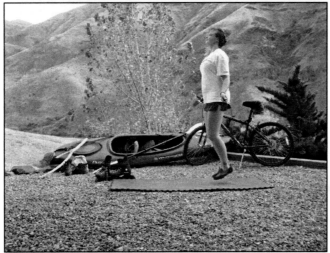

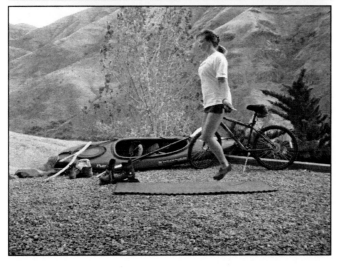

One Leg Balance with Alternating Arms

This stance with lateral arm movement is elementary but essential for balance. Stand on your right foot while raising the left foot off the ground. Extend your left arm all the way out to the side, keeping good posture and bring your right arm over your chest. Continue to balance but switch arms back and forth. For more of a challenge, put a little dip in your standing leg and rise up. Dip and rise while continuing to switch arms. Switch legs and repeat.

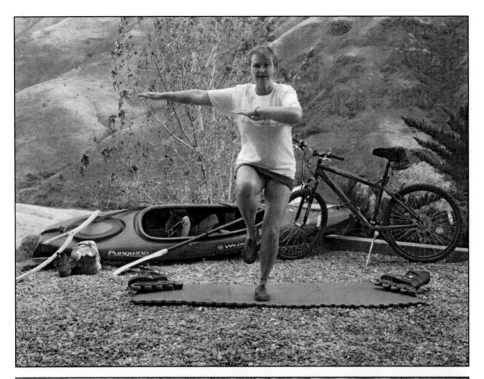

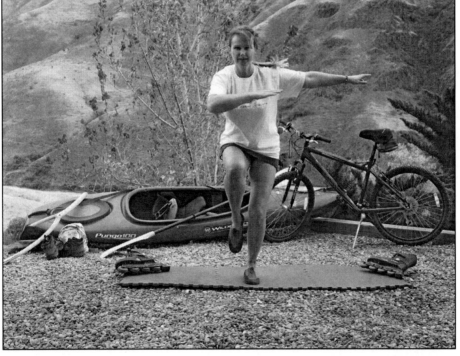

Abduction with Tubing

This balance and coordination progression comes with a bonus - abductor work. You will feel resistance in the hip and leg as you push away from the body. The tubing I am using has cuffs to place around my ankles which allows for lateral stepping and shuffling. This mimics the instability of walking or jogging in water.

Stand on left leg with hands on hips. Take your right leg out to the side, find your balance. Continue raising your leg up while pushing out laterally. Lower leg and do the same on the opposite side. When you build enough confidence with the basic action, lift your leg higher, move it backward, forward, and bring it back down. Once again, do the same on the other side. No tube? Light-weight ankle weights will do the job.

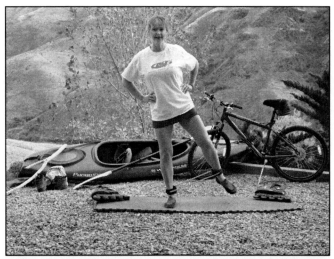

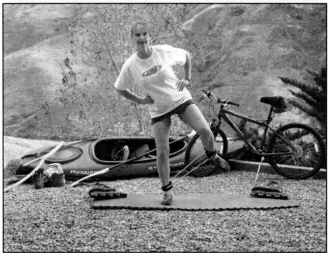

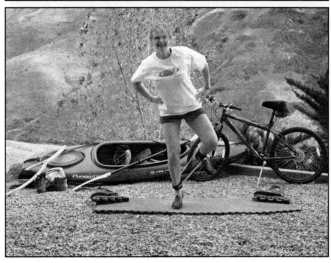

Standing Jump

In a very short amount of time, this plyometric exercise will use a lot of energy because you are increasing strength, power, and agility all at once. Bend your knees and make a half squat stance. Explode into the air by pushing through your heels. Land with soft knees when sinking back into your squat position. If you have enough space, jump forward in a hop-hop-hop fashion as well as backward.

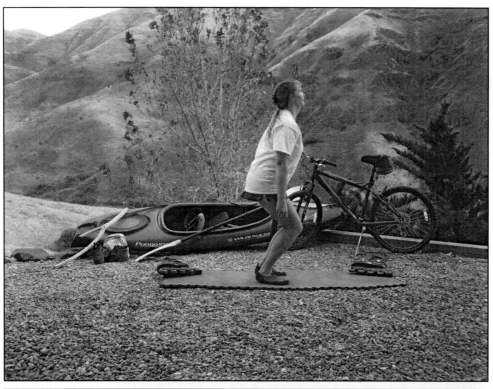

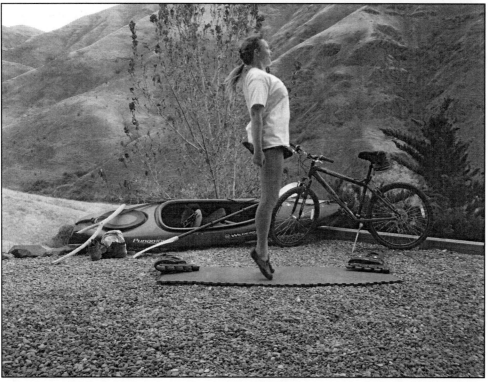

Alternating Lunge Leap

Get ready to really power it up! Stand with both arms reaching out in front of your chest. Take a big step forward and bend your knees so you're in a lunge position. Explode into the air by pushing through the heel of your leading foot and through the balls of your trailing foot. When air-bound, quickly switch feet, landing with the back foot in front and lead foot behind you. Keep soft knees when landing.

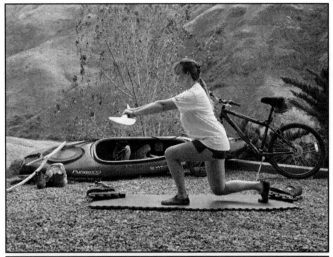

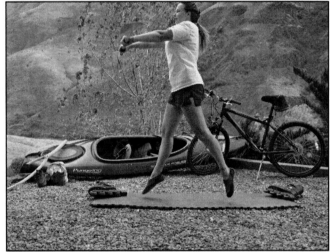

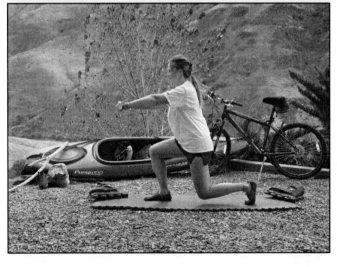

Flutter Kicks

Flutter kicks tone the core. Like crazy! Lie on your back, raise your feet up off the mat. Keep your back flat and use your arms to stabilize. Then let the fun, (or torture?), begin. Alternate fluttering your legs up and down keeping clear of the mat.

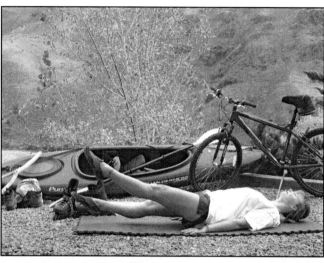

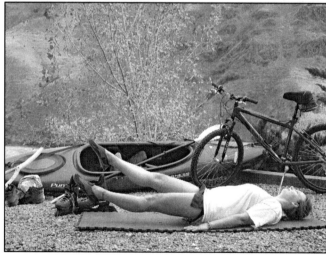

Scissor Kicks

Guess what? Scissor kicks tone the core also. Start by laying on your back and raising your legs off the floor. Spread legs wide then bring them back in. Cross one leg over the other and continue to criss-cross for as long as you want. Experiment with the distance your legs are off the ground, from a couple inches to a foot.

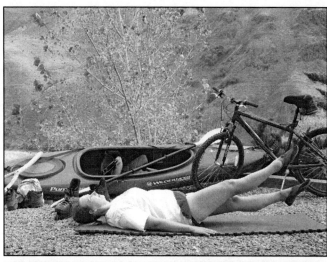

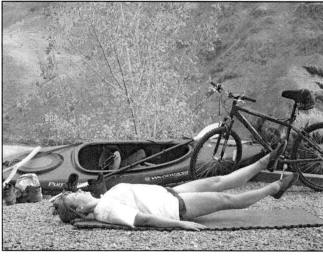

"Great job everyone, you rocked your exercise session!" I say. "Rub your muscles with warming ointment or cooling gel. Heck, put an ice pack on your neck to help you cool down. If you need more ginger, I've got it. Now we're going to shift gears and have a little R and R before tonight's rave. Follow me!"

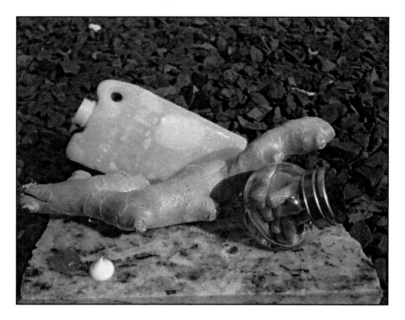

CHAPTER 4
Midday R & R

Saturday, late afternoon – early evening:

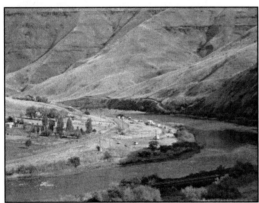 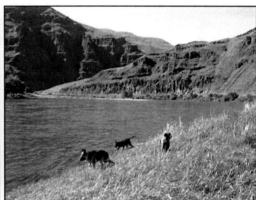

Across the street from my house down at the river, my dogs play on the bank where I meet my guests as they trickle in. The gals come from all directions and once everyone is accounted for, we start hiking through a manicured gulley up to the house. Midway through the hike, my neighbors Ray and Susan, offer zucchinis from their garden and

fresh eggs. Once at the house, the dusty or wet women change into casual wear then congregate to the front deck. On lounge chairs we sit, facing rock cliffs, watching a herd of deer traverse the cliffside trail. We sip iced tea and fruit-infused water while receiving mist from vapor misters above.

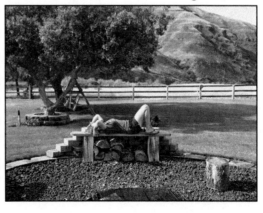

"For all the exploring and adventuring you did, how about some chill out time?"

I ask. "This midday interlude gives you a chance to take a nap, soak your feet and brush out the dog if you took one with you. You can also craft exercise gliders, which you'll be using tonight, shoot guns, and bake. Kind of like summer camp. Remember those days?"

"*Barely!*" A middle-age woman chuckles. "At least I've still got enough moxie to be running around out here having the time of my life!"

"Cheers to that!" Other chubby gals echo.

"Foot soak stations are already set up on the lower patio," I say. "There are zafus to sit on, accessories to dress the water up with items such as essential oils, Himalayan sole solution, pronounced *solay*, and dried lavender and rose leaves," I continue. "The chilled soaking water covers smooth river rocks. Rubber foot massagers for the soles are placed near the soaking buckets with a towel and mint foot finishing lotion."

After the foot soak, it is time to brush out the dogs to remove burrs, goat heads, and other stickers. The dogs are also checked for ticks and mats. Next, we cut cheap slick placemats and adhere nonslip shelving material to one side, crafting exercise gliders. We will be using these at this evening's rave.

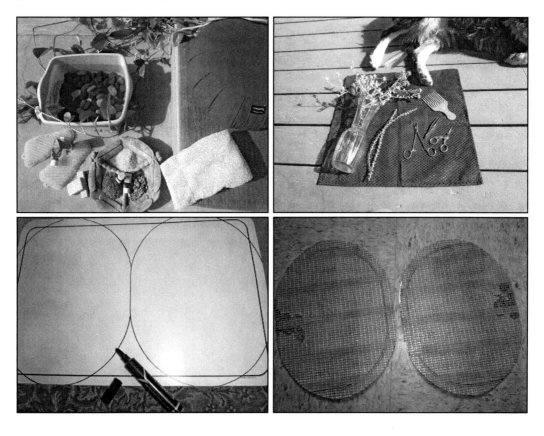

In a field behind my house are paper bulls-eye targets, water balloons, and empty beer cans placed on the ground and on platforms. I review gun safety and explain how shooting is a skill using the breath to focus. After my demonstration, I begin assisting the gals, some of whom have never handled a gun or rifle before. Many are surprised at the power of firing and jubilant when hitting a target. In the end, the ladies come out smiling as they walk away from targets strewn all over the field. They also walk away with a healthy respect for shooting.

The last activity during our midday interlude is baking bread and canning jam. We gather in the kitchen to bake from scratch, garden zucchini bread with sundried cranberries and pecans. Stations are set for grating the zucchini, measuring the dry ingredients, blending the wet and dry ingredients, and cutting parchment paper to fit the bottoms of the bread pans. When the mini pans go into the oven, the gals combine their skills to cook preserves of fresh picked plums.

"Are there any insomniacs in the group?" I inquire. "If so, meet me out in the shop."

CHAPTER 5
Recovery Rave

Saturday, PM:

Separate from the house is my husband's large shop. The industrial sized-door is raised so gals can easily follow the strobe light, glow lights, and music to my modified home dance venue. I lower the door to keep the bats out which makes the shop dark, and hand out glow sticks, glow jewlery, neon body paints, and party-size containers of magic wand bubbles.

"We are going to cap the evening off with a rave," I say. "Don't worry, this isn't *anything* like a city rave. Dancing, be it rave or Zumba, is about enjoying aerobic conditioning while loosening the body. Unfortunately, many girls and women have serious hang ups about their bodies," I continue. "Dance helps you see yourself differently. If you think you are uncoordinated and born with two left feet or you're too old or too big, then you are the perfect raver. Upbeat music gets under your skin and it moves you! Your body takes on a life of its own and your mind can forget about everything. It is movement without thought and that is beautiful."

I stand on a loft with fog rolling out of an aluminum can while techno music pulsates and clove scents the cool air.

"I will demonstrate a couple simple movements to get you started," I say. "Oh, and by the way, I will be the first to admit that I am *not* a dancer!"

Arm wave

This is a basic pop-lock move. By isolating body parts you can achieve the illusion of a wave going through your body. I can't tell you how much I like that idea! Concentrate on breaking each move down until you gain a sense of coordination and flow. When you have mastered that then speed things up to create a smooth wave-like motion.

Start with both arms out to your sides with a slight bend in the elbows. From right to left, isolate your right hand and tilt only your hand up as high as you can.

At the same time, bend your wrist forward and add a bit more bend in your elbow, raising the height of your wrist. Lower your wrist slightly below where you started and push your elbow up. Drop the elbow but raise your right shoulder as high as it will go. If you made it this far, continue. If not, it's ok to back up and try again.

Drop your shoulder but raise the left shoulder as you move to the opposite side. Drop your left shoulder and raise the elbow. Drop the elbow and raise your left wrist pointing the fingers down. Lower your wrist, unbend your elbow, then point your fingers upward.

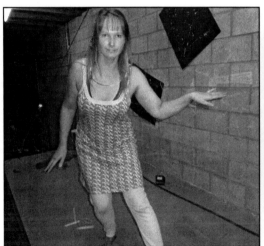 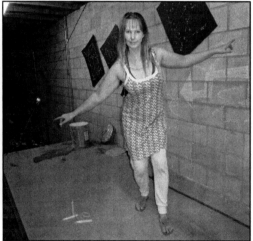

Pelvic Thrust

Work and tone those gorgeous hips and wake up that pelvis! Some women tend to have inhibitions when it comes to doing something like a pelvic thrust. There is so much power within the pelvic region that it shouldn't be ignored but it usually is. Let me help you embrace what you own with this simple instruction.

Start in a stance with slight bending of the knees. This allows for more hip and pelvic range of movement. Visualize and then mimic a hula hoop rotation with your hips. Next, remove the side to side action isolating front and back movements only. When you are comfortable doing that, increase the speed of the thrust to create smooth flowing body rolls.

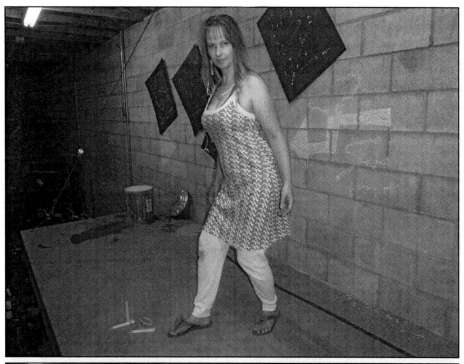

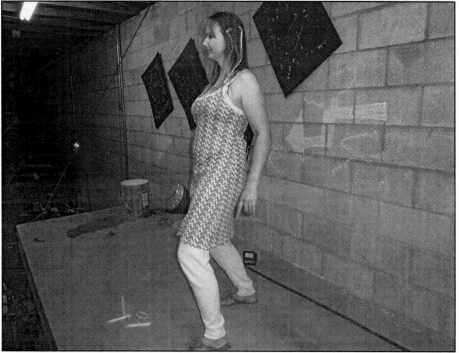

Locking Footwork

Locking footwork offers lots of attitude and uses large footwork. Let's try it! Hop on left foot, kicking right foot forward bringing your foot to knee height. Draw your right foot back and repeat. Switch feet with a hop and raise your left foot up. This time you won't bring the foot behind you but rather, follow through with a big step forward. It doesn't get any easier than that.

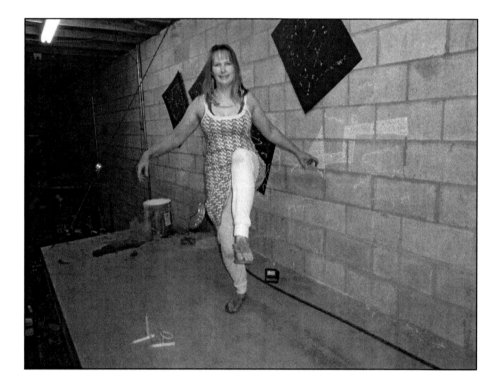

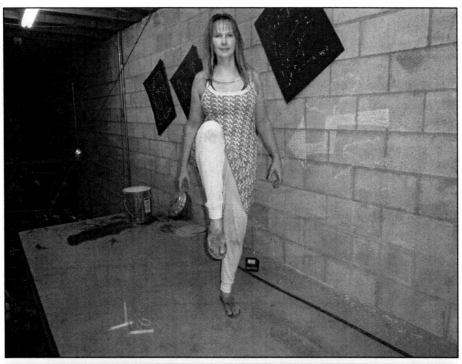

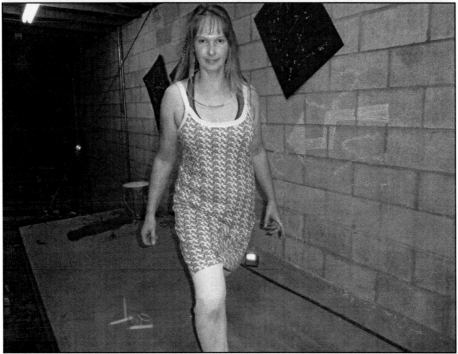

Gliding

Get your gliders out! This is an alternative way to bring your entire body into play, particularly homing in on the core, hips, and outer thighs. With limited friction between footwork and floor, you can achieve the illusion of floating. Some dancers sprinkle talcum powder on the floor for smoother traveling but you can use your crafty gliders instead. Variations to gliding include floating and sliding. When a dancer travels with a toe-to-heel movement similar to moonwalking, the technique is called floating. In contrast, sliding is just like it sounds. Like sliding on ice. Who hasn't done that? Gliding incorporates a push-pull where you can push forward, pull backward or push-pull in circles. This exercise is improvisational so you can move any direction you want. What I'm demonstrating is a side-to-side forward glide.

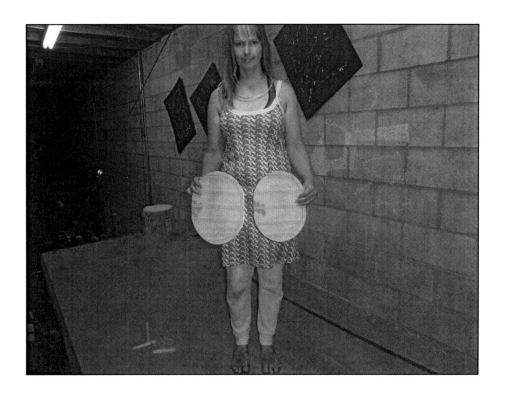

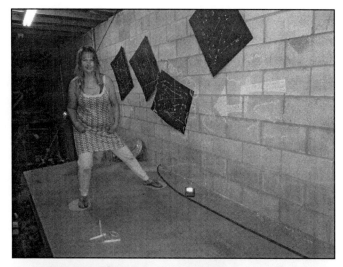

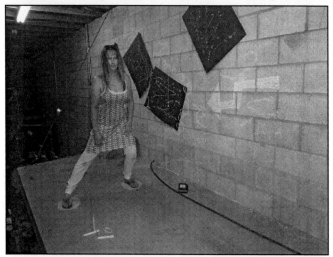

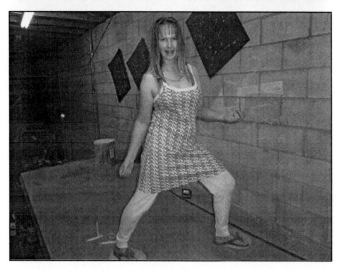

Leg Drain Against a Wall

Lower yourself down on to the floor near a wall and get into a seated position. Sit facing the wall then scoot sideways up against it as close as you can. You may find it easier to scoot on a bath towel or blanket. Bring both of your legs up against the wall by lowering your back horizontal on the floor. In this passive position you can allow your feet and legs to take a well-deserved break. Enjoy the relaxation for at least a few minutes or longer.

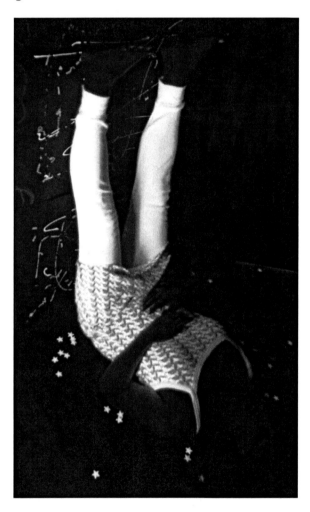

Never feel guilty about closing yourself off from the world to rest. Resting is not a crime! Sneak in a power nap if you're short on time. Taking a nap is great medicine for your entire well-being and it helps an active body recuperate. If I were president, there would be rest stations at every worksite. Wendy for president!

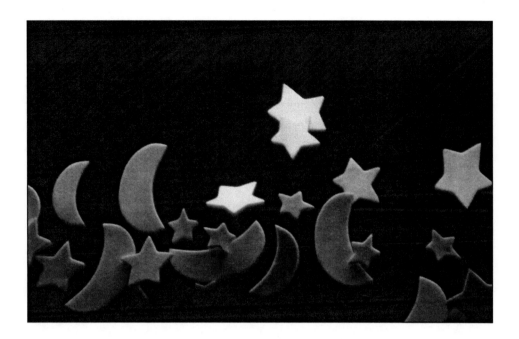

What do raver's eat? Ravers tend to snack on munchie foods like fruit smoothies, fruit cups, popsicles, lollipops, and Pixie Sticks. Just make sure the snack has the potential to glow!

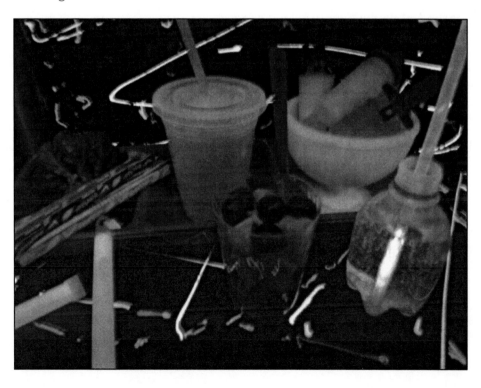

CHAPTER 6
Working Homestead

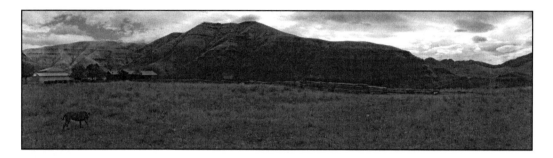

Sunday, AM:

"This is the last day of your weekend exercise getaway," I announce. "The previous two days were pretty casual. Just the way I like it and I'm sure you agree. Casual and fun, those *were* the days! We covered a lot of activities with a ton of variety. But, I want to make sure you get your money's worth before you head back home. I am going to let you in on some hearty exercise that is the real deal out here.

"Do you recall me saying, when it's time to work it is *time to work*?" I continue, "well, my dear friends, I wasn't kidding. It would be a shame not to allow you the experience of tending to the hands-on labor intensive activities required out here in the summer. Even though I don't live on a ranch or on a farm, I still live on sixteen acres of land that has to be kept up. There is grass to mow and water, trees to climb, prune, shake out, and water."

We stroll around the perimeter of the house as I keep talking.

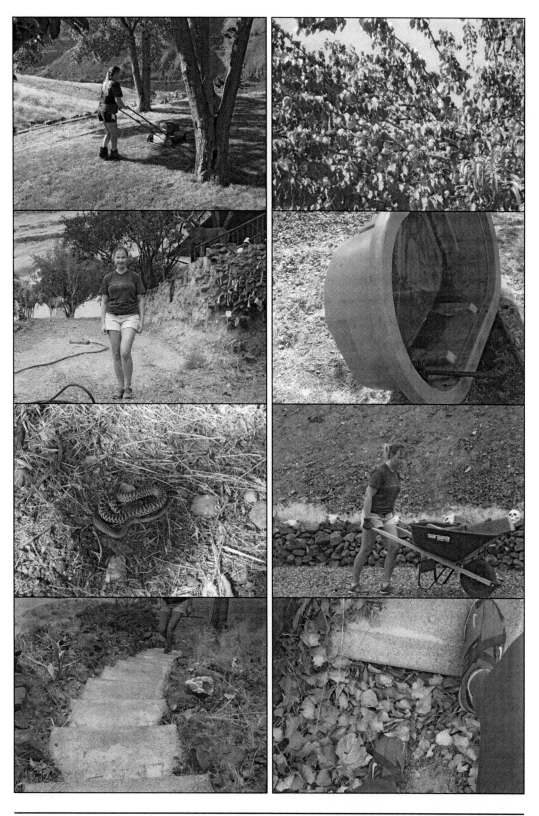

"There are tubs to scrub so animals have clean, fresh water available to them. There are snakes to jump from, wheelbarrows to push, stairs to climb, leaves to rake, and ropes and hoses to pull and haul. If there is too much foliage or too many dead leaves near the house that can create a fire hazard. Snakes and fire are the two things Clayton and I go out of our way to avoid." I lead the group to the kitchen.

"A busy day of chores starts with a hearty breakfast for sustenance and energy. Forget about Red Bull. My con pana with a splash of Carolines or kalua will get you buzzing like nothing else!" I say.

We all pitch in and cook a breakfast buffet which is taken out and eaten in the orchard.

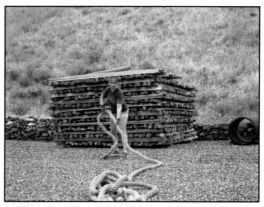

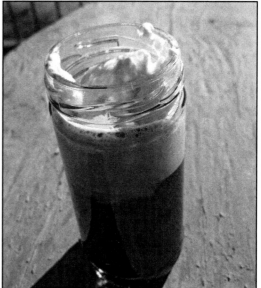

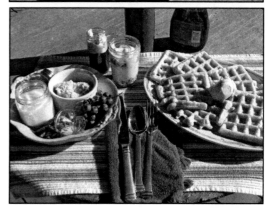

"Today's fitness session focuses on functional training with dynamic balance and coordination exercises," I say. "Strength and power, speed and agility, and endurance exercises are included in the mix. This combination will help prevent fatigue so you can get the job done." I wander over to a rebounder.

"Go ahead and start your warm up with little health bounces. You don't even have to lift your feet off the surface," I instruct. "Baby bounces get the lymph flowing through your system which helps flush out junk. After a few minutes, make bigger jumps."

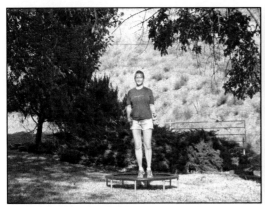 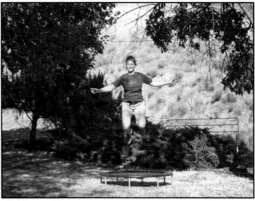

"With acceleration and deceleration forces on the body, rebounding works its magic on a cellular level," I explain. "One of the benefits is detoxing one's system through the lungs, skin, and lymph. Digestion improves, not to mention balance and core strength, and you get an endorphin boost. Rebounding is ideal for warming up or cooling down and it's perfect for aiding with recovery. None of the jumps have to be out of this world since simple bounces have as much benefit as big jumps. Big jumps are much more exciting though!"

Wrist strengthening

It is not a bad idea to increase wrist strength. A good indicator signaling wrist weakness is if you find they get sore when doing push-ups. The first exercise is for you to pick up a dumbbell, then bend wrist forward and backward as far as you can. Your palms can face up like the picture shows or down. Doesn't matter to me as long as you can actively bend the wrist. The second exercise is moving your hand side to side rather than up and down. These wrist exercises can be done throughout the day.

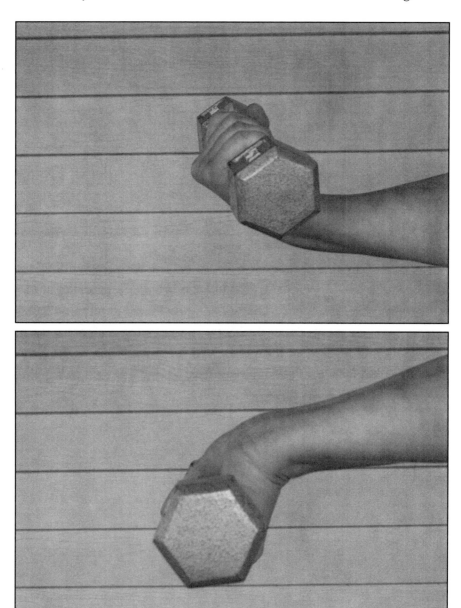

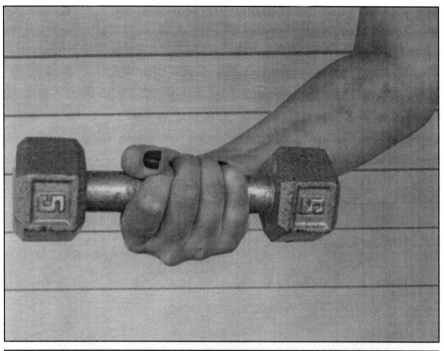

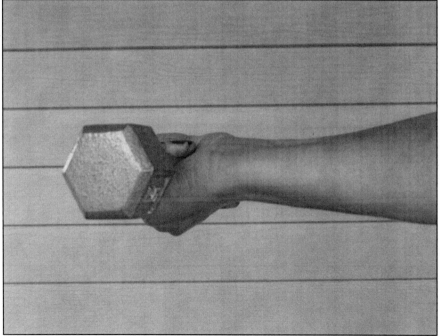

Dumbbell Chest Press

Lie on your back on a bench, exercise ball, or elevated platform. Whatever it is, make sure your feet touch the floor and your head and neck have something to rest on. If your head's about ready to snap off backwards then you're positioned wrong. With a dumbbell in each hand, position your arms like I'm doing here. They don't have to be perfectly aligned at 90-degree angles, just hold the dumbbells steady to the sides of your chest. Slowly push both hands up to the sky and straighten the arms. Your palms and fingers face away from you as they would when you wave hi to someone. Without weights, of course! Bring 'em down. Then push up and keep doing this. You want to feel the chest working.

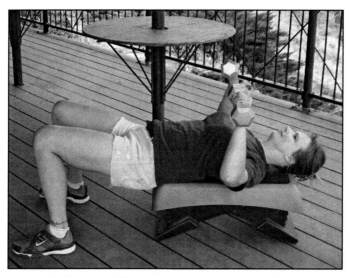

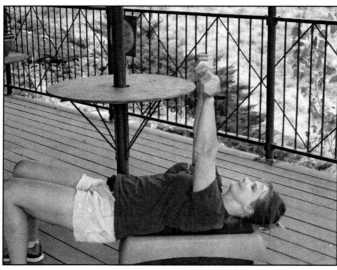

Standing Bent-Over Row

Grasp a set of dumbbells and turn your palms in so they face each other. With feet about shoulders width apart, squat a bit and lean forward slightly. Knees do not pass the toes. If they do then put more weight on your heels to shift you back. Allow for a small arch in your lower back and find a spot in front of you on the ground to stare at. Pull both dumbbells back like you're pulling a big sack of potatoes without any help from your husband because he's watching TV. Do it like you mean it and really stick your chest out. At about this point, you should feel the shoulder blades squeeze together. Perfect!

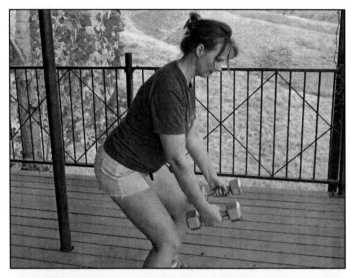

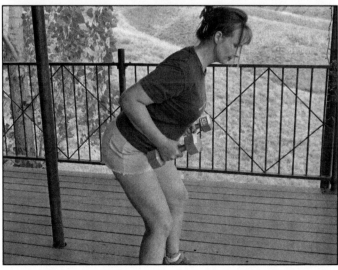

Dumbbell Deadlift

You can do this with straight legs if you want. Mine are bent because I wasn't thinking about it at the time. Straight or bent, the choice is yours. Don't say I never give you choices, eh! Have a set of dumbbells on the ground, placed about hip width apart to the outer sides of each foot. With knees bent, or legs straight, and back straight, bend down at the hips to grasp a dumbbell in each hand. Keep your head facing forward as you extend hips to standing position. Keep your legs tight and squeeze your butt when coming up.

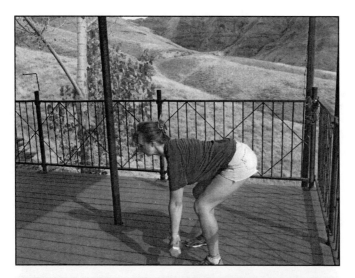

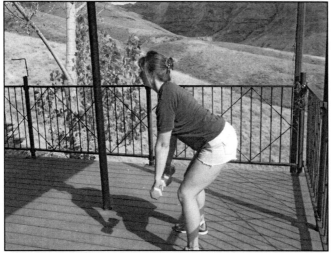

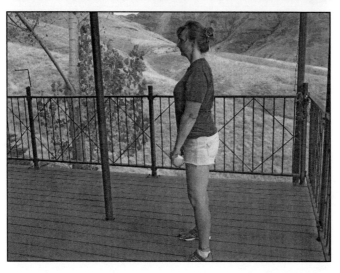

Sissy Squat with Alternating Hammer Curls

Find a wall or tree to squat against, with a pair of dumbbells in your hands. See how my arms are positioned? Do that. And while you're holding the dumbbells and squatting against something, think of the dumbbells as hammers. You've hammered a nail once or twice in your life and that exact movement is what you'll do here. One controlled hand at a time. Wrists do not bend. Wrist and forearm are a single unit. Alternate hammering.

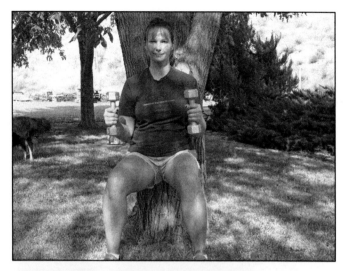

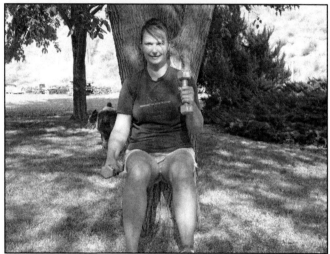

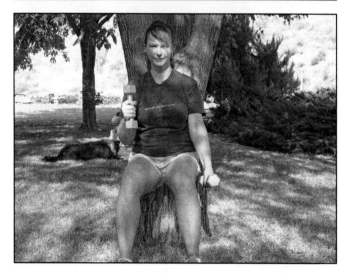

Triceps Bench Dip

This triceps exercise is cool because it works your shoulders and upper back, not just the triceps. Strong wrists work well for bench dips and here's why. You are going to bend your arms and lower your body, then push yourself back up to the starting position. You will be supporting your weight on your arms and that will translate to your wrists. Don't sink so low that your shoulders start feeling unnaturally pulled back though.

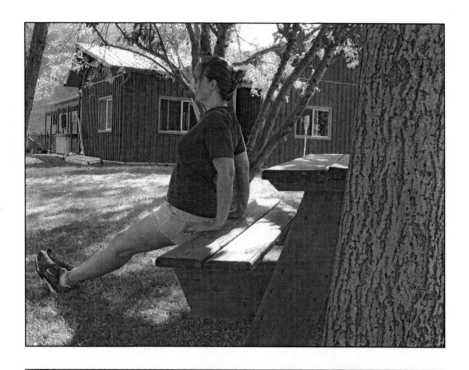

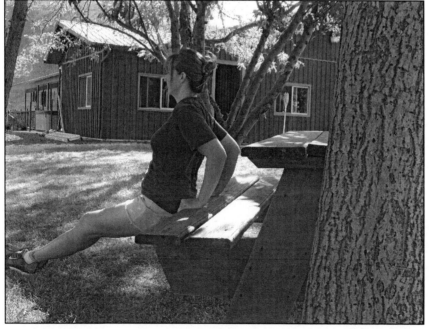

Rocking Horse

Grab a set of dumbbells, keeping both arms straight down. Lean forward on your right foot while lifting your left leg behind you. Rock back on your left foot, lifting the right leg so that your thigh is parallel to the ground in front of you. Switch legs and repeat sequence on opposite side.

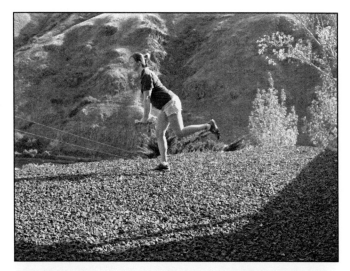

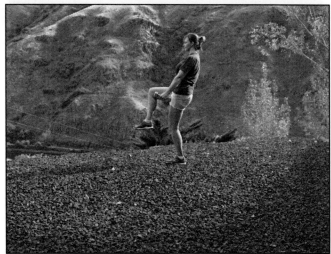

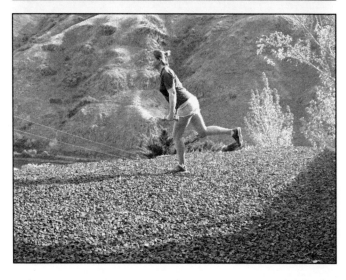

Berry Shuttle Run

Why on this good earth would anyone want to do a berry shuttle run? Because it beats another boring session on the old hamster wheel, (i.e. treadmill, elliptical, stationary bike). My grandma's friend crocheted the strawberries and grandma sent them to me from Canada. They were to go in the cute glass bowl, also sent by grandma, and placed on a shelf to admire. I came up with a better use for these wonderful berries and bowl. It is the shuttle run!

I found a stretch of patio to do this on and the way I get going is to dump the berries at random on one end of the patio. I walk or jog to the opposite end with basket in hand and set the basket down on the pavement. Then the game begins! I run-jog-skip-speed walk to the scattered berries, squat down to pick one single berry up, and bring it back to the basket. The berry must go in the basket but if I miss, I still have to pick it up making sure it gets in that darn basket. Then I keep doing this back and forth shuttle until all the berries are in the basket. After allowing for a short break, I dump all the berries out once more and repeat the shuttle a second time. And as many times after that as I want.

If you don't have a hamster wheel or a whole lot of room for endurance type activities, the shuttle may be the perfect alternative. Be creative and use pebbles or coins instead of strawberries and a tin can instead of a glass bowl. Challenge yourself against a timer for a little more heat!

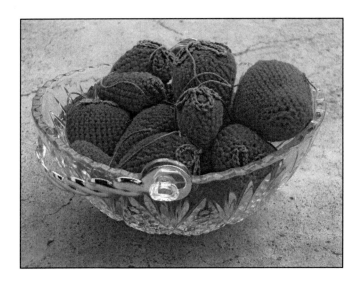

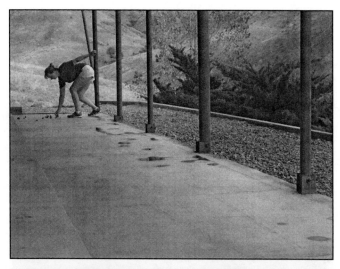

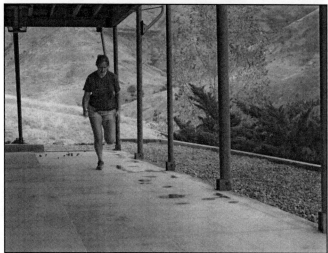

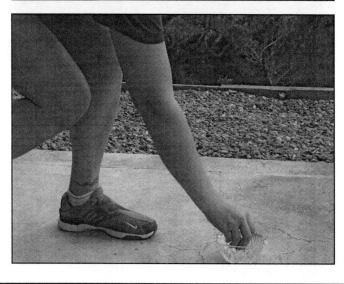

Towel Shake

Get a big ole towel, grab the corners of one end, and raise your arms allowing the towel clearance from the ground when you shake it out. Shake the thing until your shoulders sting which tends to come sooner than later. This is a perfect example of muscular endurance at work.

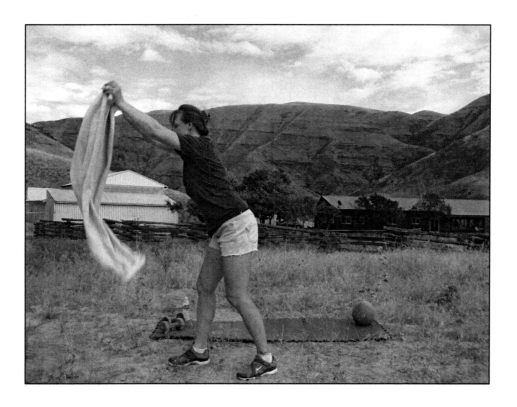

Med Ball Slam

Jack, the ball-loving border collie, did not get hurt in any of these ball exercises. With that said, the ball slam is a play with power. If you think you aren't very powerful, go slam a medicine ball into the ground. And do it over and over again. If the ball bounces back up, snag that sucker but if it doesn't, squat to get it. To really drive the ball, start by holding it above your head.

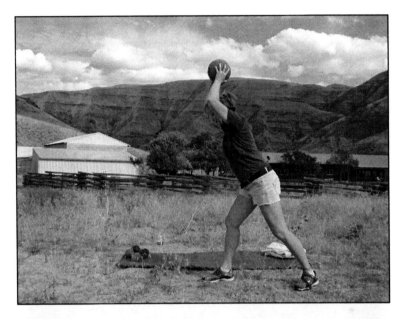

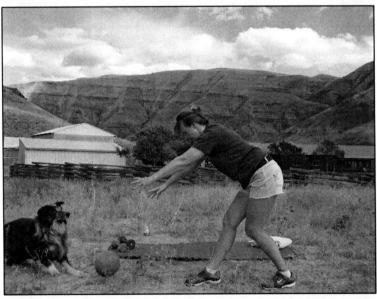

Wood Chop with Med Ball

Hold the medicine ball the way I'm doing here. Look at it like Jack is and then pretend you're chopping wood by bringing the ball across your body, ending near the opposite knee. Unlike the ball slam, you want to keep a hold of the ball with both hands so you can reverse the motion and come back to start with a controlled swing.

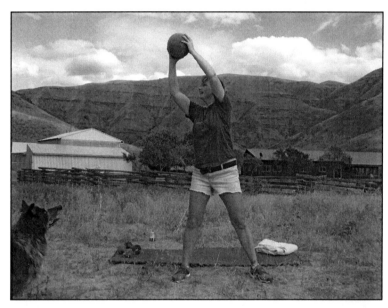

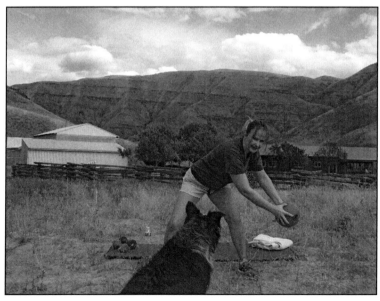

Squat Press Up

Ok gals, pick up a pair of light to medium dumbbells and hold them at about shoulder height. Your palms should naturally face forward and your elbows flare out to each side. This encourages you to stick the chest out and tighten your belly. Sit back into a squat or partial squat, if you have knee issues. Push up through the heels and, at the same time you come to a standing position, raise both arms above your head. Come back to a squat with dumbbells settling in the shoulder region. Similar to the medicine ball using many muscles at once, this compound movement does the same.

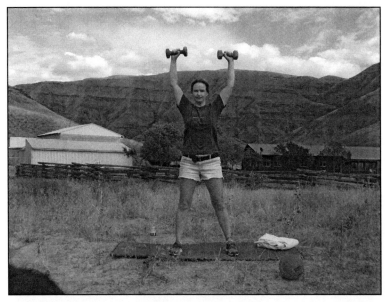

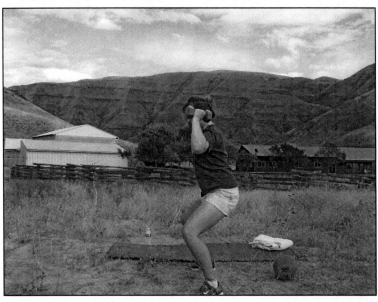

T-Push Up

Start in a push up position, grasping a dumbbell in each hand. Easy enough! Unfortunately, the hard part is the next step. Come on down as far as you can without sinking your lower back. I know, it's hard to tell how your back looks when you can't see yourself. If you suck in your gut and think about bracing for a punch, I'm pretty sure your lower back will straighten out. Hold that thought…

Now, slowly start to turn your body to one side and raise *that* hand up to the sky. The foot connected to your top leg should lead the foot that's attached to your lower leg. Don't think too hard about the choreography because your feet will fall into place quite naturally to accommodate the body as it does its little twisting action. Voila, madam, you got it!

Twist back down to start. Guess what? Time to do the other side. Don't think about your lower back sagging. Now that I mentioned it, I know you will think of your lower back sagging.

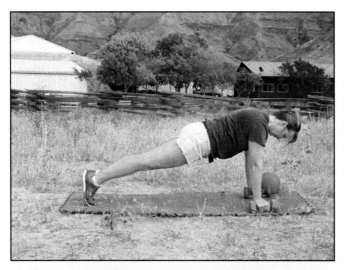

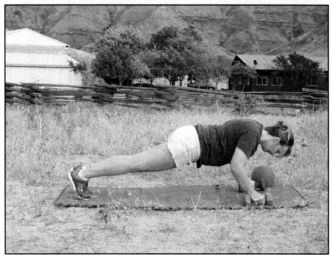

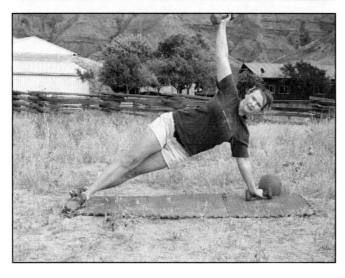

Pullover Crunch with Medicine Ball

Lie on your back on the floor or a mat holding your arms straight above your chest. In your hands you will have a medicine ball or a single dumbbell held at both ends. Bend your knees and keep both feet up in the air. Congratulations, you now look like a dead bug! Tighten the belly before simultaneously reaching the ball overhead and extending one leg. Keep your foot off the ground six inches to a foot, I don't care. As long as the foot is in the air, you're fine. Then come back to dead bug and repeat the movement but push out the opposite leg this time.

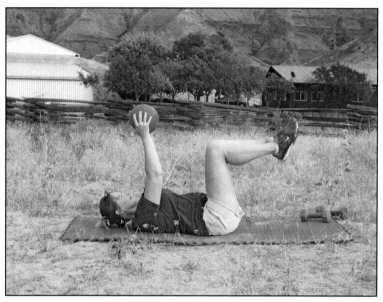

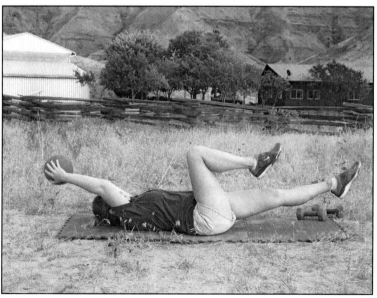

Charlie's Angels

Sit on a mat leaning back at a slight angle. You will feel your abs kick in, I promise. If you want to, go ahead and squeeze a medicine ball between your feet, otherwise keep your feet on the ground. Make a pistol with your hands then twist to one side and pause to shoot. Twist to the other side, pause and shoot. Oh, don't forget to smile because you love your obliques and you feel them loving you back!

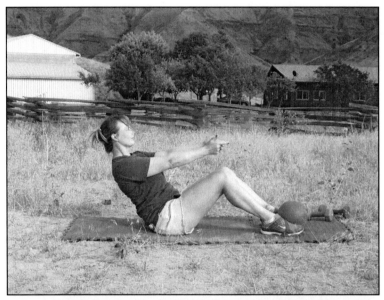

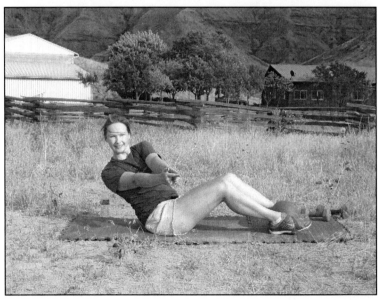

"Nice work!" I say. "You completed the last set of exercises for this weekend getaway."

"A hard day on the homestead is better than an easy day at the office," a gal comments. I smile and nod in agreement.

"Doesn't it feel good to turn things up every once in a while with higher intensity exercises?" I ask. "In addition, compound movements complement your daily activities, especially when you have to do physical work. Okay! The work is done. Now it's time for some cheap entertainment!"

Cheap Entertainment:
Soak in Tub and Watch Jack Chase Ball!

Fill tub with cold water, get in, and watch the dog chase after an unwanted and soon to be flat stability ball.

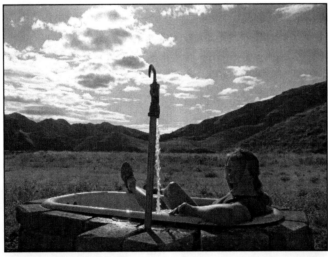

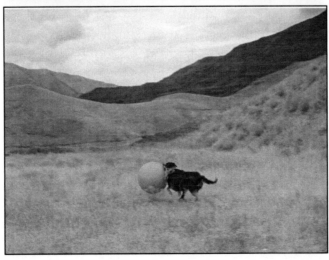

CHAPTER 7
Until Next Time

Sunday afternoon:

After my guests pack their things, I meet them at the door with gift boxes.

"Chubby gals, you entered Hells Canyon and explored what it means to exercise recreationally," I tell them. "For that, I applaud you. Hells Canyon isn't such a scary place after all, and exercising shouldn't be either. I dare say, under the right circumstances, it's a lot of fun!" I hand a box to each gal.

"I want to send you off with a small gift," I say. "Within every gift box is a fresh-baked mini zucchini loaf with cranberries and pecans, paired with a jar of your homemade plum preserves, and a spreading knife. There's also a set of sun and sand scented votives, and my collection of weekend exercise getaway recipes."

The gals express their gratitude with hugs.

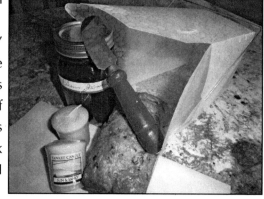

"Let me warn you ahead of time," I pause before continuing. "The recipe measurements are only guestimates because I tend to wing it in the kitchen. If something you make within these recipes isn't quite up to par, don't be afraid to tweak it. And don't say you weren't warned!" I laugh.

The gals laugh too, and promise to stay in touch with me and each other through facebook and my blog at www.wendystrack.com.

"This may be the end of our weekend exercise getaway but that doesn't mean we still can't be friends," I comment. "I hope you had as much fun as I did. Until next time, take care and please come visit again soon!"

Wendy's Collection of Guestimated Recipes:

If you recall, on Friday during the jet boat tour, lunch included falafel in pita pockets with cucumber-mint raita, lentil salad, a lemon bar, and herbal iced tea. The mildly spicy falafel was nicely counter-balanced with the cool raita. This sandwich was perfect for picnicking in hot weather.

Falafel in pita pockets with cucumber-mint raita

4 servings (about five 1-inch balls per serving)

<u>Falafel</u>

½ cup yellow split peas
¼ cup dehydrated vegetables (onion, potato, garlic, carrot, peas, parsley)
1 cup canned garbanzo beans, rinsed
½ cup onion, chopped
1 clove garlic
1 to 2 tablespoons fresh lemon juice
1 teaspoon each ground cumin, coriander, chili powder
2 egg whites
½ cup dry breadcrumbs
Oil for frying
4 pita pockets
Spinach or other hearty salad greens, washed and dried
Lemon wedges

Prepare the yellow split peas according to package directions. Reconstitute dehydrated vegetables in warm water for about 15 minutes, drain if needed. While the peas cook, puree the garbanzo beans, onion, garlic, lemon juice, and spices. Add and pulse the egg whites and breadcrumbs, then incorporate the reconstituted vegetables and cooled, drained peas.

Heat an inch of oil in a pan on medium-high. Scoop the falafel with a small ice cream scooper to make little balls, binding them with your hands. Set the balls in the oil, leave to cook for about 1 minute each side. When the entire surface has browned remove falafel from pan and drain on paper towel.

Make the raita. To build the sandwich, cut the pita bread in half, stuff the halved pockets with spinach or salad greens then place 4 to 5 falafel balls inside the pocket. Top with raita and squeeze with lemon, if desired.

Cucumber-Mint Raita - about 4 servings
½ cup plain soy or coconut yogurt
½ teaspoon fresh squeezed lemon juice
2 tablespoons fresh mint leaves, cut into small pieces with kitchen scissors
3-4 tablespoons cucumber, peeled, seeded and thinly sliced

Mix ingredients together with a spoon.

The briny-ness of the olives marries well to this earthy grain-based salad. This lentil salad is ideal served room temperature or even on the lukewarm side after the marinade has a chance to soak in.

Lentil Salad with Marinade - 4 servings

Lentil Salad
½ cup cooked brown rice
1 cup canned brown lentils, rinsed
1 tablespoon olive oil
¼ cup onion, chopped
¼ cup each carrot and celery, thinly sliced
2 tablespoons of either fresh spinach, cut in thin ribbons or parsley, chopped
1 clove garlic, pressed
2 pinches celery seed
1 shake of garlic salt
Coarse black pepper
6 stuffed green olives, sliced
2-3 tablespoons olive brine

Heat olive oil in a pan over medium-high. Add onion, carrots, celery, spinach or parsley, garlic, celery seed, garlic salt and black pepper. Leave uncovered allowing to cook until vegetables are barely tender, 10-15 minutes, stirring occasionally. Add rice, lentils, olives and brine, mixing everything together turning heat to simmer. After a couple of minutes, remove from stove and set aside to cool. Prepare the marinade.

Lentil salad Marinade
3 tablespoons olive oil

2 tablespoons balsamic vinegar

1 tablespoon French mustard

1 teaspoon dried tarragon

½ garlic clove, crushed

Whisk all ingredients together. Mix marinade into lentil salad. Cover and refrigerate for at least a few hours. Serve room temperature.

Nothing says perky like a tart lemon bar full of fresh-squeezed lemon juice. Coconut flour used in the crust gives a subtle sweetness with a hint of coconut aftertaste. The bars look nice because they are dusted with powdered sugar after cooling off and just before serving. Personally, I like the lemon filling so much that I usually double the batch and bake it longer. Worth the wait!

Lemon Bars – 9 bars

Crust
½ cup unsalted butter, room temperature

¼ cup powdered sugar, sifted

½ cup flour

½ cup coconut flour

Filling
1 ½ cups sugar or more to taste

Zest from 4 lemons

¾ cups fresh squeezed lemon juice (about 4 lemons) or more to taste

1 teaspoon baking powder

4 eggs

Powdered sugar to sprinkle

Heat oven to 350 degrees. Lightly grease and flour an 8 x 8 inch glass baking pan. On high speed, mix butter and powdered sugar then add the flours ¼ cup at a time until dough binds. When the dough comes together, press into pan, bake 20 minutes or until the surface begins to brown slightly. Remove from oven.

Beat all ingredients for the filling, except powdered sugar, on high speed until it mixes together. Pour over crust. Bake for about 40-45 minutes until there is no indentation when touched in the center. Take out of oven and cool on wire rack. Before serving, cut into bars and sprinkle with powdered sugar.

After a day on the river you returned to Tiki Hut Lounge for a light dinner. A must-have at any shindig are small bites loaded with big flavors. Tiki Hut Lounge served those up with an exotic spin that was even on the healthy side. Friday night's menu included tuna-pineapple kabobs, basmati rice, cod chowder with an Asian twist, and mango with lime. We had so much fun!

Tuna-Pineapple Kabobs over Steamed Basmati Rice – 4 servings

Marinated Tuna Kabobs
1 cup teriyaki marinade
1 pound albacore filet, cut into 1-inch cubes
Fresh pineapple, cut into chunk sizes for skewers
Olive oil for drizzling

In a large Ziplock freezer bag put both the marinade and albacore cubes in to marinate; refrigerate at least an hour. Remove tuna from the marinade, stab with skewers alternating with pineapple chunks. Prepare basmati rice according to package and/or steamer directions.
Preheat grill or broiler, drizzle skewers with olive oil. Place on broiler pan in oven for 2-3 minutes each side. Serve over rice.

Cod Chowder with an Asian Twist ain't your momma's chowder!

Cod Chowder with an Asian Twist – serves 4-6
1 to 1 ½ pounds cod, rinsed, gently squeezed, reserving juice
2 – 3 teaspoons pureed lemongrass from prepared tube, (you can find prepared herb and spice blends in the produce section at most grocers)
1 – 2 tablespoons pureed ginger from prepared tube
2 tablespoons green curry paste
1 cup clam juice

¼ cup soy sauce

2 tablespoons brown sugar

1 ½ cup canned coconut milk

1 cup coconut milk (milk alternative)

Tomato, chopped

Green onion, chopped

Cilantro, chopped

Lime wedges

3 cups steamed basmati rice

Cut the cod into 1-inch chunks and set aside. Lightly sauté lemongrass, ginger, and green curry paste until blended then add clam juice, soy sauce, brown sugar, coconut milks, and cod with reserved juices. Cook over medium-high heat stirring frequently for about 5 minutes. Simmer uncovered on low heat for a ½ hour. Stir tomato, green onion, and cilantro into simmering chowder and let heat up for a couple minutes. Serve over basmati rice and squeeze with lime.

Speaking of limes, the absolute only way to eat a mango is with fresh-squeezed lime juice. This simple addition elevates the mango flavor to another dimension. Peel the fruit, cut it horizontally around the pit then into vertical sections. Pare individual sections away from the pit, placing them in a bowl and squeeze lime juice over the flesh. Enjoy!

If you are a meat eater then sausage and bacon aren't just for breakfast anymore. Salmon isn't just for dinner either. Saturday morning we walked to the neighbor's house and ate breakfast on his lovely river beach. If you have a cast-iron pan, pull it out because this will contribute to the salmon searing beautifully. Be careful not to overcook the flesh, as it will keep cooking once it's removed from the heat source. This recipe utilizes the broiler instead of a campfire.

Seared Salmon – serves 4

4 salmon filets, rinsed and dabbed dry

2 - 3 tablespoons cooking oil

Turn broiler on high. Set pan on rack and let heat up about 10 minutes. With an oven mitt, carefully remove pan and drizzle oil to cover entire surface. Place under broiler for another 2 to 3 minutes. Take pan out and set on a wire rack then lay the filets in the pan leaving them to fry. If the cuts are thick, cover the fish with a lid so they will cook through faster. After frying 5 minutes on one side, turn the filets over and let cook another 5 minutes. When inner flesh is not transparent any longer it is ready to plate.

Serve with sweet potato chips and eggs.

Sweet Potato Chips – 4 to 6 servings
    4 sweet potatoes
    Ice water
    Cooking oil
    Salt

Peel each potato and slice wafer thin. Set slices in a bowl of ice water as you continue peeling and slicing. While preparing the potatoes, heat about ½-inch cooking oil in a large pan on medium-high. When you're done prepping the potatoes, grab a huge handful from the water, shake excess water off, then dab slices dry with clean kitchen towel. Carefully set one layer at a time in the oil, which should sizzle gently. Fry for 3 minutes each side. With slotted spoon remove the potatoes from the oil, drain on paper towels and salt. Serve with ketchup if desired.

I am all about eating dessert first, like for breakfast! We enjoyed a generous piece of strudel with our healthy sidekick of salmon and eggs. Here is the recipe.

Apple Strudel - 8 slices

Pastry and Filling
    5 baking apples, peeled, cored and sliced
    ½ cup sugar
    ½ teaspoon of each, cinnamon, cloves, nutmeg
    ¼ cup raisins or currants
    1 tablespoon flour
    Juice from 1 small lime or lemon
    8 sheets filo pastry
    1/8 cup butter, melted
    1/3 cup cream cheese or cream cheese alternative, if desired

Topping
1 tablespoon each, sugar and cinnamon

Icing
¼ cup powdered sugar, sifted
Vanilla beans scraped from the pod
1-2 teaspoons coconut milk

Heat oven to 400 degrees. Line baking sheet with parchment paper. In a large bowl combine the apples, sugar, spices, raisins or currants, flour, and juice. Set aside. Brush each sheet of filo with melted butter, stacking layer upon layer until all the sheets are greased.

If using, spoon dollops of cream cheese or cream cheese alternative on the surface of the dough, staying away from the edges. Next, spoon the apple filling in. Gather the edges of the filo and gently roll like a burrito, tucking both ends under. Place the seam side down, brush with melted butter, sprinkle cinnamon sugar on the top.

Bake for 20 minutes then rest strudel on wire rack. While strudel is cooling prepare the icing in a small bowl by stirring together all the ingredients. Drizzle on strudel once it has cooled.

Saturday afternoon lunch took place wherever you found yourself in the Chief Joseph Wildlife Area. The best lunch to take along in the field is one that isn't going to break out all over and make a mess in your backpack and it must keep well in any temperature. The humble but classic peanut butter and jelly sandwich is *it*. Sure, it might get squished but the pb and j still tastes good and provides an excellent source of energy. No one is ever too old to enjoy a peanut butter and jelly sandwich. Adults might prefer gourmet butters, such as almond or sunflower, though.

Energy bars, cheese and crackers, and small candies are convenient snacks but so are vegetables. Lemon cucumbers are small and juicy but carrots and celery are good too. Coconut water should be a staple in any pack because it replenishes electrolytes without artificial sweeteners. Coconut water is an acquired taste!

Saturday evening we ate late at the modified rave exercise party. As you noticed, food for a rave doesn't have to be anything near entrée status. Keep it simple with cool snacks using common ingredients. Berries, maraschino cherries, and pineapple come together for a fruit cup, mold popsicles out of juice you've got in the fridge, pull out the hard candy and Pixie Sticks, and wash everything down with bubbly water like seltzer or club soda with citrus twists. Be creative and throw in some glow in the dark or neon straws! If your snacks glow under a black light then that turns your simple nibbles into a fun conversation piece. Here's a recipe for a fruit smoothie that will make you pucker.

Tart Cherry Smoothie – 2 to 4 servings

1 cup cranberry juice
1 cup vanilla yogurt
1 cup frozen cherries
1 teaspoon citric acid powder
Handful of crushed ice cubes

Combine all ingredients in a blender and process until smooth.

Sunday morning came quick but we took our time waking up to breakfast on the homestead. Plan on making a mess in the kitchen and don't plan on cleaning up until after you've eaten, drank, rested, and done did your chores on the outside. Then you can come inside and start cleaning the kitchen, that is, if you feel like it. Or put it off until the cows come home.

Cake Waffles – makes about 8 servings

2 eggs
2 cups cake flour
1 cup milk
¾ cups half and half or whipping cream
½ cup melted butter
1 tablespoon brown sugar
3 teaspoons baking powder

As waffle iron is heating, put all the ingredients in a blender and blend until smooth. Let batter sit for about 5 minutes. Spray non-stick oil on waffle iron then pour some batter on the hot iron and close the lid. Bake until steaming stops and remove the waffle. Stack waffles on a large serving dish as they cook and keep warm in an oven set on lowest temperature. Serve with syrup and butter.

Oatmeal Wendy's Way – 4 servings

3 ½ cups water
2 cups oatmeal
1 tablespoon brown sugar
1-2 tablespoons real maple syrup

Boil the water, stir in oats, bring oats to a rolling boil, then reduce heat to medium. Cook about 5 minutes, stirring occasionally. If there is still liquid, turn stove to a simmer and let oats sit a while longer. If all the liquid is absorbed, stir in the sugar and maple syrup. Put a lid on the oats and turn heat off. Serve with sides of coconut or almond milk, currants, pecans or sunflower seeds, brown sugar, and granola.

Coconut Yogurt Parfait with Granola – 4 servings

4 cups plain or flavored coconut yogurt
2 cups prepared granola
Agave syrup

Alternate yogurt and granola in pint size jars. Top with agave syrup.

Some mornings when I know I have a lot of work to do, I get going with straight espresso topped off with thick homemade whipping cream. And a splash of big girl liqueur. You will need a coffee grinder and an espresso machine to make this bittersweet concoction.

Con Pana – 1 serving at a time

Double espresso
Whipped cream
Irish cream or Kahlua

Grind beans into a fine texture and scoop into your portafilter, then tamp the grounds. Pull between a double and quad shot of espresso. Top with generous dollop of whipped cream and drizzle with Irish Cream, Kahlua or other choice of liqueur.

Sunday afternoon was time to say goodbye. Going away boxed goodies contained road food worth reminiscing over.

Zucchini Bread with Cranberries and Pecans - 4 mini loaves

   3 cups shredded zucchini
   1 ½ cup sugar
   2 teaspoons vanilla
   3 eggs
   1 cup wheat flour
   2 cups white flour
   2 teaspoons baking soda
   1 teaspoon each cinnamon, cloves
   ½ teaspoon baking powder
   ½ cup dried cranberries
   ½ cup pecans, chopped

Heat oven to 350 degrees. Spray sides of baking pan with oil, put parchment paper on the bottom. Mix sugar, vanilla, and eggs. Slowly add flour, baking soda, spices, baking powder, and zucchini. Stir in cranberries and pecans. Put batter in pans, using a spatula to spread to the corners. Bake 40-45 minutes, or until toothpick inserted in center comes out clean. Cool 10 minutes on wire rack in pans. Loosen sides of loaves and remove from pan. Set bread bottom side down on wire rack to finish cooling.

Plum Preserves – makes 8 half pints

   4 ½ cups plums, washed, pitted and chopped with skin
   ½ cup water
   2 ¼ cups sugar
   1 pack pectin
   Pint jars

Boil plums and water stirring consistently. Reduce heat to medium-low, cover and simmer for about 5 minutes. Add the sugar bringing to a boil again, stirring constantly. Add pectin, boil 1 minute and don't stop stirring! Remove from stove and skim off the top layer of film. Pour preserves into jars, secure the lids and boil to make a seal.

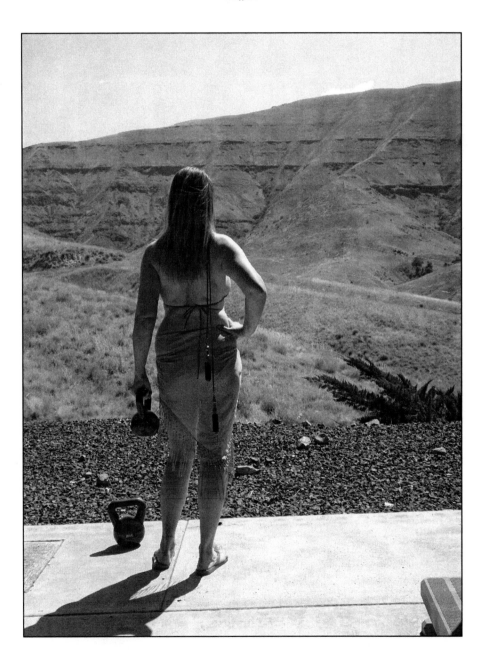

APPENDIX A
A Few Yarns about Hells Canyon

The Hells Canyon geography is an imposter to North America. The impressive 8,000 – feet of rock was, at one time, under an ocean when western Idaho used to be a *coastline*. Fossils cemented within the limestone, which formed in the ocean, came from coral reefs from a location similar to the South Pacific. In addition, high in the cliffs are large pillow formations resulting from lava flowing a mile *beneath* the ocean.

Within a ten mile distance the Hells Canyon terrain goes from 7,000-feet in Oregon, drops down to 1,500-on the Snake and climbs back up to over 9,300-feet in Idaho. Extreme? Yep. As a result of the extreme landscape, Hells Canyon is abundant with prime big game animals.

Wooden boats of the 1900s filled with supplies ran downriver on the Snake and were never heard from again. A monstrous waterfall located between the vertical canyon walls existed before Hells Canyon Dam was ever erected and ate wooden boats and their crew for breakfast, lunch, and dinner. Now the monster is buried in a watery grave behind the dam.

Speaking of monsters, Nez Perce tribal legend tells of a good mythical figure known as Coyote. Coyote dug Hells Canyon with a big stick to safeguard the tribe's ancestors in the Blue Mountains of Oregon from the "Seven Devils" across the gorge in Idaho.

Definitions for scenic and wild regarding Hells Canyon National Recreation Area: *Scenic* is more settled and has road access. Motorized vehicles are allowed. *Wild* does not have roads and the only mode of getting to this part of the country is by foot, horseback, helicopter, (depending on access), or floating.

Hells Canyon is home to the largest free-roaming elk herd in the United States.

During the summer at lower elevations you might see an odd snake called a rubber boa. It's odd because it doesn't seem to have a head. The rubber boa only gets about 14 to 30 inches in length.

The number of rattles on a rattler snake does not tell how old the snake is in years. As the rattlesnake ages parts of the rattle become lost.

APPENDIX B
Some Safety Stuff

Taking care of yourself in the heat:

- Pack plenty of water.
- To maintain blood volume and core temperature, avoid dehydration when exercising out in the heat. Drink 1 cup fluids every 15-20 minutes. Carbonated drinks don't count when trying to rehydrate. Stay off the booze until you return to a safe oasis.
- Bring sunscreen, lip balm, sunglasses and hat for protection.

Wild animal and plant precautions:

Cougars:

Don't hike or engage in a solitary activity, especially during the twilight hours. Cats can see you very well and they tend to hunt at this time. Go in groups and carry some form of protection whether it is a large stick, mace or a pistol. If you see trees used as a scratching post or a fresh kill barely buried, keep on walking. If you stop to check it out you could get more than you bargained for. If you come upon a cougar, give it an escape route. If the cougar appears to threaten you, stand tall, wave your arms and scream to appear like a threat and not prey. Do not run from a cougar and do not fall to the ground faking "dead." It won't work.

Bears:

Bears are fast! If you notice bear scat along a trail make plenty of noise. A pocket fog horn is ideal for flushing critters out of brush giving them an opportunity to get away from you. If you are face to face with a bear don't stare it down and do stay calm. Act in a passive manner. If a bear bluff charges you, do not run. Rather, stand your ground allowing the bear to walk away. If the bear does approach you, then fight by kicking, punching, and throwing rocks.

Rattlesnakes:

You might hear the rattlesnake before you see it. Until you do get a visual, do not move. If you have a long stick, probe around you cautiously. If you don't have a stick, then look very carefully. When you have the snake in view, slowly back away from it but make sure you know what you're backing into. You don't want it to be another snake. If you get bit do not suck or cut the wound. Do remove any constricting jewelry or clothing to prepare for the swelling. Keep bite area below the heart. Your buddy should run for help. If you are alone, hopefully you have a 2-way radio to make contact with someone since cell phones do not work out here.

Poison ivy/poison sumac:

Wear a protectant barrier if you go down by the water. If you do make contact with the plant(s) don't scratch and try not to contaminate more areas of your body or clothes. The sappy juju is very prolific and you will be miserable for weeks if you do not contain and treat it immediately.

Other stuff to know:

- Carry a radio in your group.
- Be prepared to care for the feet, human and dogs, as there are nasty non-native weed species that will poke, stab, and insert themselves into anything that comes in contact with them.
- Make sure there is goop in your bike tires or you will get a flat.
- Remember to wear your life vest.
- Know your boundaries if you are not familiar with this rugged territory.

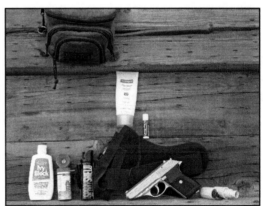

About the Author

Wendy Strack, not your typical fitness author, lives in southeast Washington with her husband, Clayton, and their dog, Jack.

If you enjoyed *Chubby Gal Fitness: weekend exercise getaway,* you'll get a kick out of what's coming in *Old School Fitness: weekend retreat for bad girls.* One can only imagine…

Please visit www.wendystrack.com today!

CPSIA information can be obtained at www.ICGtesting.com
Printed in the USA
BVOW021932270612

293802BV00003B/2/P